Grow It Heal It

Natural and Effective Herbal Remedies from Your Garden or Windowsill

Christopher Hobbs and Leslie Gardner

RODALE.

© 2013 by Christopher Hobbs and Leslie Gardner

Rodale books may be purchased for business or promotional use or for special sales. For information, please write to:

Special Markets Department, Rodale Inc., 733 Third Avenue, New York, NY 10017

Printed in the United States of America

Rodale Inc. makes every effort to use acid-free ♾, recycled paper ♻.

Cover and still-life photography © 2013 by Sandra Johnson with prop styling by Anthony Albertus:
iv, vii, viii, ix, 106, 113, 116, 123, 129, 135, 142, 146, 149, 151, 153, 159, 160 (3), 166, 168, 169, 171, 173, 178

Plant photography:
Courtesy of authors: 6, 18 (top), 18 (bottom), 22, 26, 28, 30, 36 (left), 36 (right), 38, 42, 44, 48, 52, 58, 60, 62, 66, 70, 72, 80, 82, 84, 88, 96, 98, 100, 102

© istockphoto: 2, 24, 32, 34, 50, 54, 64 (left), 64 (right), 68, 74, 76, 86, 90, 92 (left), 155 (left), 167

© Rodale: 16, 40, 78

© Steven Foster: 4, 8, 12, 14, 20, 56, 92 (right), 94, 154 (2)

Book design by Carol Angstadt

Library of Congress Cataloging-in-Publication Data is on file with the publisher.

ISBN 978-1-60961-570-3   paperback

Distributed to the trade by Macmillan

2   4   6   8   10   9   7   5   3   1   paperback

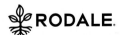

We inspire and enable people to improve their lives and the world around them.

rodalebooks.com

I would like to dedicate this book
to my family—my partner, Leslie Gardner,
and son, Ken Hobbs—as well as all the
herbalists past and present whose experience
with healing plants and love of nature has
inspired me and lighted my path.

—*Christopher Hobbs LAc, AHG,*
PhD candidate (UC Berkeley)

In gratitude, this book is dedicated
to my roots and shoots: my parents, Robert
and Ruth Gardner, who make the world a
better place; my beautiful Goddess, Diana;
my dear Christopher and Ken; and the ancient
lineage of herbalists in every page.

—*Leslie Gardner MH, AHG*

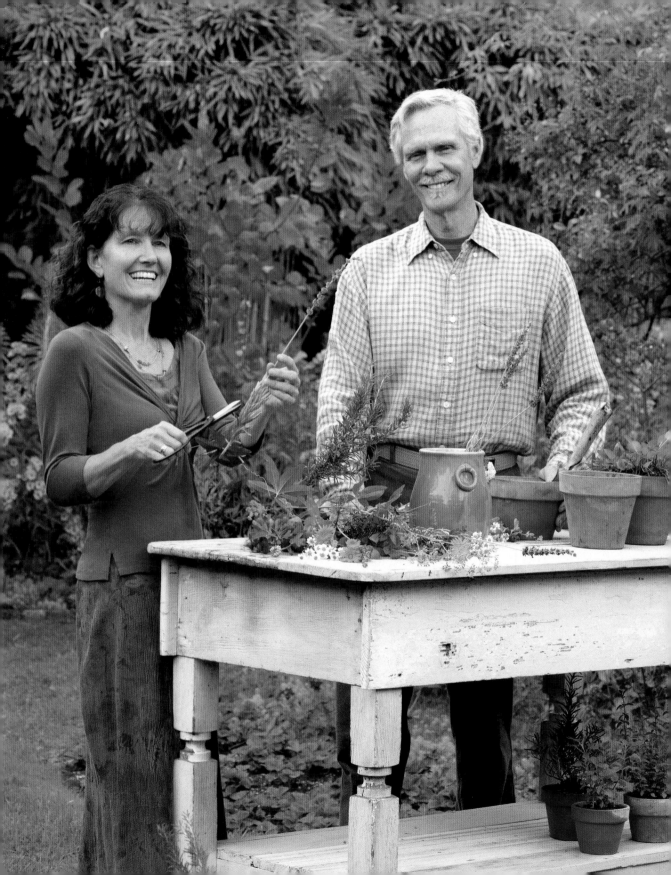

CONTENTS

INTRODUCTION

Safeguarding health and healing have always been human concerns, and for at least 5,000 years, people have been creating herbal preparations to treat illness and discomfort.

How do we know? Fragments of what were likely medicinal plants and flowers have been found in archaeological digs that uncovered Stone Age fire sites. The Sumerians, who in the 4th millennium BCE resided in the area that is now Iraq, left written records of medicinal herbal preparations that are strikingly similar to those we use today. And the healers of ancient Egypt built a sophisticated body of knowledge about herbs and their uses that became the basis of modern medicine. In this, the Egyptians surpassed the Greeks, who embraced the practice of using diet, healthy living habits, and other natural methods to treat disease and preserve health 3000 to 1550 BCE (5,000 to 3,500 years ago).

We find the same evidence of the ancient use of herbal medicine in Asian cultures, where Ayurveda and traditional Chinese medicine have been practiced for thousands of years. The ancient herbal knowledge of the Sumerians, Assyrians, Egyptians, Greeks, and Romans was passed on through the writings of Hippocrates, Pliny, Galen, and especially the physician Dioscorides. Dioscorides lived in the 1st century CE and wrote the most long-lasting and influential herbal of all time: *De Materia Medica* (meaning "of medicinal substances"). Dioscorides was a physician in Nero's army and travelled with the Roman legions for many years, and his book was the ultimate authority on herbal practice for 17 centuries! *De Materia Medica* was translated into Persian in the 7th century, which brought this ancient wisdom into North Africa and the Middle East, and later into the first European medical schools in Italy between the 10th and 13th centuries. From here, medical knowledge traveled northward throughout Europe over the next few centuries. It is said that the first printed book was the Bible, and the second, an herbal. Many households had these two books on the mantelpiece for centuries to come.

All of the great herbalists of the Renaissance—Turner, Fuchs, Brunfels, Dodoens, Parkinson, and the "King's Herbarist," John Gerard—wrote large works that are still known and studied by today's herbalists. They are rich and colorful in their language and are an indispensable record of the human use of healing plants through the ages to that time.

Herbalism continued to be used both as folk medicine and in the professional medical trade through the 17th, 18th, and 19th centuries, culminating with the American Physiomedicalists and Eclectic Physicians, who presided over their own medical schools and journals. These traditions produced several renowned books, most notably the 1902 edition of the *King's American Dispensatory*, which is still well known today and is available online.

By the 1930s, however, the medical standard was turning toward synthetic drugs as replacements for herbal preparations, although the use of herbs continued in some areas. In the United States, the 1936 edition of the *National Formulary*, a record of drugs prescribed and sold in pharmacies, included numerous herbal extracts such as echinacea, saw palmetto, dandelion, blue cohosh, and Oregon grape root.

Most herbs were dropped in later editions, and by 1995 only a few remained. Fortunately, the art of growing medicinal plants in a home garden and making teas and other herbal preparations is alive and well in many countries around the world today, as it has been for many centuries. In fact, an "herbal renaissance" (as it has been called by Dr. Paul Lee, a Harvard divinity professor who launched one of the earliest large American herbal gatherings) began to flower in the late 1960s. The famous herbalist Dr. John Christopher was traveling extensively in the United States at that time, teaching good old-fashioned herbal medicine. He promoted his favorite herbs, cayenne and lobelia, and was arrested numerous times for "practicing medicine without a license."

In the late 1970s, Rosemary Gladstar founded the first American herbal school, the California School of Herbal Studies, as well as the first national herbal conference at Breitenbush Hot Springs, Oregon, in 1981. From there, a new generation of herbalists began meeting, teaching, and practicing herbalism throughout the country, and many are still active today.

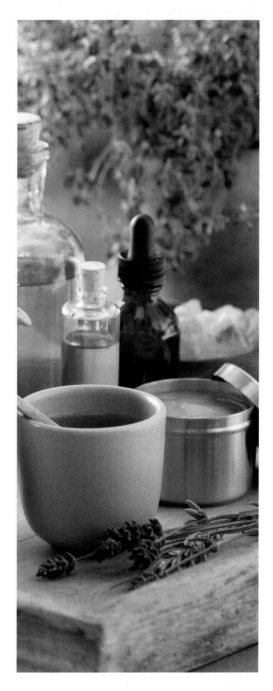

You can join the ancient and modern tradition of empowered self-care and exploration by reading and using *Grow It, Heal It*. You, like ancient healers, hold in your hands a record of remedies that reaches back through the ages. You can grow and nurture plants that heal, just as they did. The preparations you make using the herbs from your garden or windowsill can help to ease pain, preserve health and vitality, and promote long life. And, like those who have gone before, you can gather this healing power, prepare it, and use it for the comfort and improved health of yourself and those around you.

Safety

What about the safety of the herbs themselves? Science has revealed much about individual plant constituents. Some, such as caffeine, have been thoroughly studied. Today we increasingly understand the subtle effects of many herbs on cellular metabolism and the tissues and organs of the body. When scientific studies are done, the effectiveness of herbal preparations is typically consistent with a given herb's history of use, as long as the herb is prepared and taken in accordance with its action and safety. And when herbal treatments are compared to treatments with pharmaceutical drugs, fewer and milder side effects are recorded for the herbal remedies. In addition, herbal preparations are nearly always less expensive than pharmaceuticals. Although scientific study has not yielded conclusive research on the safety and efficacy of every popular herb, it has confirmed a good deal of traditional herbal practice and established many excellent reasons for using herbs for healing. In this book,

we've distilled the results of numerous human scientific studies of herbal remedies, and we've shared our decades of direct experience with herbs in the garden and in the wild, as well as in clinical and scientific settings. Like all medications, some herbs can be harmful when misused or taken carelessly. Your individual physical condition and current medications can bear upon which herbs you should take and which you should avoid.

Planning Your Herbal Medicine Chest

When you're choosing which herbs to grow and use at home, take a look at the current contents of your medicine cabinet. Most people keep a supply of pain relievers, cold medicines, digestive remedies, something to promote sleep, and products for wounds, rashes, or burns. Prescription drugs may be in there, too. You can grow herbs and make simple and easy products at home that can treat most of your everyday medical and health issues. Within these pages you'll find remedies for injuries, respiratory tract infections, digestive upset, undesirable symptoms that might arise during menstruation and menopause, and even safe herbal teas to ease nausea and other symptoms associated with pregnancy. Although you can purchase herbs to make these recipes, it is so much more exciting and meaningful to grow and harvest your own. Your appreciation and awareness of the beauty and healing essence of herbs growing in your garden (and in their natural homes in the wild) are the starting points for a lifelong journey and a healing relationship with plants. We often say that it is only by growing herbs that you can really know them as medicines and fully understand their power and effectiveness.

Growing a Medicinal Herb Garden

Not so long ago, the only medicine available came from herb gardens or wild land. By the Middle Ages and the Renaissance, the increasing sizes of cities made herbal medicine gardens quite practical, and a tradition was born. Sometimes communities cooperated to grow a medicinal garden. Nearly everyone worked in the gardens, and many families made their own handmade medicines. So you see, it's almost a certainty that you come from a long line of herbalists, in one form or another! You can pick up the thread of your ancestors and rediscover the pleasure and satisfaction that comes with being self-sufficient in your own health care, while delighting your senses at the same time. An herb garden need not be large, but it should suit your personal needs for healing. Do you lead a hectic life with too much stress? Consider a calming garden filled with chamomile, lemon balm, wild lettuce, and California poppy. From such a garden could come delicious fresh teas, tinctures to settle your nerves and bring on sleep, and dried calmatives to last the winter. If cold weather seems to be one long ordeal of colds, sniffles, flu, and congestion, try a garden of echinacea, elder, garlic, lemon balm, peppermint, thyme, and yarrow; they will provide antiviral action, boost your immune system, fight congestion, and reduce fever. Within these pages, you'll discover that many medicinal herbs grow happily in pots, making a traditional garden unnecessary. Container gardening, an old art that is gaining in popularity once more, is particularly suitable when you don't have access to a sunny garden patch. A few pots can yield useful medicinal herbs for a variety of ailments. When purchasing plants and seeds for your garden, be sure that you choose the medicinal variety of the particular herb you're seeking; closely related plants may differ significantly in their medicinal properties. You'll want to pay special attention to the guidelines we give for each herb in the Know It chapter. Plant names can be confusing, too. If you have trouble finding correct varieties or species, check our Resources listings.

Above all, use your time with the plants as an opportunity to develop your creativity, your intuition, and your individuality. The art and science of herbalism is your birthright, and you can breathe life into the knowledge in these pages only by putting it into practice. May your garden be bountiful and your medicines bring only the best to you and yours!

—*Christopher Hobbs*
—*Leslie Gardner*

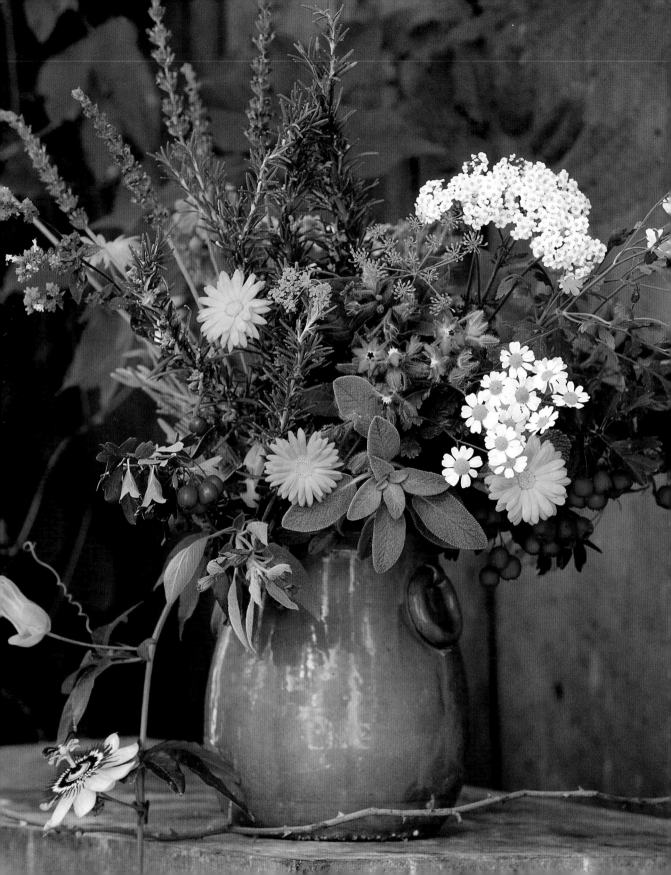

PART 1

Know It

Welcome to the world of plant-based healing. Meet the 50 herbs—from aloe vera to yerba mansa—that you can grow to help relieve or treat symptoms you experience with short-term illnesses, minor injuries, or chronic conditions. You'll also discover how you can use many of these herbs (as well as some common weeds) as part of a daily regimen for vibrant health.

Aloe vera

Family: Xanthorrhoeaceae

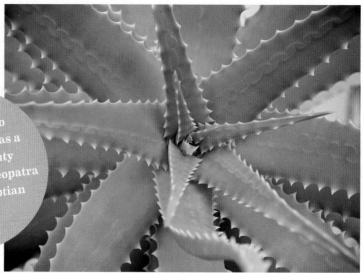

According to legend, aloe was a favored beauty treatment of Cleopatra and her Egyptian court.

Aloe vera

This miraculous first-aid remedy should be on every windowsill, deck, and patio! Originally hailing from Africa, this succulent has been cultivated since antiquity. In fact, there are no known wild stands of aloe anywhere in the world. But that's all right—we know where it lives.

Description

Aloe is a multiple-leaved succulent, and those thick, fleshy, green leaves are the main attraction. Sometimes the leaves are spotted with white, and their margins are variously serrated with white, curved, thorny teeth. The yellow and red flowers appear erratically and usually bloom after a mild, wet winter followed by a warm, dry spring. Aloe will not survive a hard freeze, so most of us have to grow it indoors or grow it in a protected spot outside and bring it inside for the winter.

Preparations and Dosage

Although many products are available, such as creams, salves, lip balms, and bottled gels, nothing works as well as the fresh gel scraped or squeezed right from a leaf (apply the gel several times a day, as needed) or the freshly drained juice. For the many various products available in markets, follow the directions on the labels.

Healing Properties

The thick gel from inside aloe leaves can be applied to any kind of skin trauma, including burns, stings, bites, acne, scrapes, and wounds. This gel contains glycoproteins and polysaccharides shown in studies to speed the healing of burns and wounds and stimulate production of new tissue. Quite a few preliminary laboratory studies show that aloe can speed the healing of wounds, burns, herpes sores, psoriasis, HPV lesions, seborrheic dermatitis, and frostbite when compared with silver sulfadiazine cream, a standard pharmaceutical treatment. One study summary concluded that wounds treated with aloe healed up to 9 days faster than those treated with a placebo cream. It has also shown promise for aiding glycemic control in diabetics and for reducing high cholesterol levels. Though aloe studies are of mixed quality, an overall assessment shows clear benefits. We recommend using aloe gel right from the leaf (or a commercial product that is labeled "100 percent aloe vera gel") for healing wounds and burns, and also for soothing rashes and sunburns. Aloe can also be applied to your face and skin to counteract dryness with mild irritation.

Aloe is worth trying for gum inflammation, mild to moderate gum disease, mouth sores, and trauma after dental work.

Safety

Aloe leaf is the source of two types of products. The first is derived from the resin directly under the skin, and it has stimulant laxative properties. The second is the inner gel, which is not laxative and is used for drinks and body-care products.

We recommend against the use of aloe gel during pregnancy or while nursing unless it's used under the advice of an experienced practitioner.

In the Garden

Aloe is ideal for a rock garden or xeriscape (low-water or desert area). Hummingbirds love the flowers! It won't survive a harsh winter, but if you only get a few mild freezes, it will grow outdoors with just a little cosmetic damage each winter. Give it well-drained, sandy soil (such as a commercial cactus and succulent mix) in a big pot, and place it in a sunny, warm spot. Poor drainage will cause the leaves to shrivel and blacken; give it a rest in the winter and don't water it! If this deer-resistant plant is happy, it will develop side shoots, which can be gently separated from the mother and repotted. These will take up to 2 years to reach full size.

Harvesting Aloe Vera: For the gel, slice off the tip of a leaf and apply the mucilaginous open interior to burns, bites, and itchy spots. You can further slice the removed portion lengthwise and expose more of the gel. For the juice, wait until the leaves are 1 to 2 feet long, and don't remove more than three or four leaves from a plant at a time. Cut them cleanly, close to the plant, and immediately stand them upright, cut side down, on a support or sloped frame. Place a container underneath to catch the juice as it drains out. Bottle and keep the juice refrigerated.

Andrographis paniculata

Family: Acanthaceae

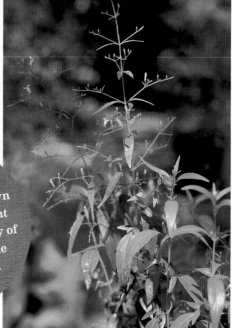

Andrographis was the only known malaria treatment until the discovery of quinine from the cinchona tree.

Andrographis

Known in India as the "king of bitters" and in Chinese herbal medicine as *Chuan Xin Lian,* andrographis has only recently become available in the West. The herb does live up to its name as wickedly bitter, so you'll find it sold in capsule and tablet form, singly and in formulas. Although it may not top your list of tasty culinary delights, you will be won over by its long list of clinically documented antiviral and immune-boosting effects. The aboveground herb is most often used today, and, less commonly, the root or whole plant can be used.

Description

The plant is erect and widely branching, reaching 2 to 3 feet tall, with long, green, square stems; small, lance-shaped leaves; and tiny, flecked, white to pale pink flowers in long, slim clusters. In its native tropical India and Sri Lanka/ Southeast Asia, it grows in patches in moist, shady locations from plains to hilly areas, roadsides, and fields.

Preparations and Dosage

You will probably find this herb most palatable in the form of tablets or capsules (take them one to three times daily), but traditionally it has been prepared as a tea or a decoction, often with a sweet herb like licorice or stevia to counter the bitter flavor. Take 1 to 2 teaspoons several times daily, sipping it before meals to take advantage of its digestion-enhancing effects. Start with a weak tea and work up to a stronger dose, especially if you like bitter tonics.

Healing Properties

Andrographis is famous for its ability to protect us against infections, both viral and bacterial. Western herbalists are increasingly recommending it as a top herb for preventing and helping to shorten the symptoms of colds and flu, and clinical research supports this use.

Some years ago, while in rural Thailand, we were shown this herb by the village herbalist, who said, "I want to show you the most famous herb in Thailand." He pointed to andrographis! It turned out that every pharmacy we went into had bottles of andrographis prominently displayed. It is widely recommended in both Ayurveda and traditional Chinese medicine for infections and for regulating blood sugar, and scientific studies have shown it to have liver-protecting and digestion-promoting actions, among others.

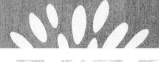

Safety

Andrographis is considered a generally safe herb and has a very long record of use in both Ayurvedic and traditional Chinese medicine. Long-term use at a high dose (two to three times what is recommended, or higher) can lead to digestive upset or skin rashes in sensitive individuals. We recommend sticking with the label recommendation, especially for products containing high concentrations of standardized extracts, where the product label specifies the level of one group of active compounds, the andrographolides. For your garden-grown and dried herb, you can take up to 1 teaspoon of the ground powder daily. Use this herb with caution during pregnancy—especially early pregnancy.

In the Garden

In India, this herb is cultivated during the rainy season, although we've found it to be quite adaptable to drier climates, if reliable irrigation is provided. You'll need a nice, long growing season, and that means that in all but the most southern zones, a greenhouse or sunny indoor porch is a good option. (If you're planting outside, andrographis should do best in full sun to partial shade.) Since the structure is so diffuse, clump several plants for a nice effect, and make sure to fertilize them with compost and manure or a seaweed or fish emulsion preparation. Start them from seed (easiest) or cuttings, or even by layering, in the best conditions. Andrographis will be free of insects and diseases, but the seeds will need warm soil to germinate and then will take 3 months or more to mature to their best medicinal potency. In very warm climates, they can sometimes overwinter and go a second year, but in most climates, you'll experience these plants as annuals.

Harvesting Andrographis:

Cut the flexible, smaller stems and leaves during the flowering stage—in warm climates, you could get a small second flush of growth. The very thin stems dry quickly, but remember to check the largest sections of the stems to make sure that they are "crackly" dry so they won't mold in storage.

Angelica archangelica

Family: Apiaceae

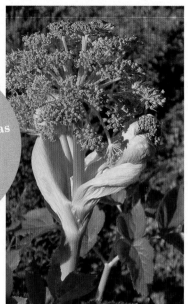

A favorite of all herb gardeners, this aromatic herb was included in secret medieval elixirs and digestives.

Angelica

This angel of the garden is legendary in European tradition. During the time of the Black Death, the archangel Raphael reportedly revealed to a monk that this plant was the cure for the plague, and to this day villagers in outlying areas of northern Europe wear it as a magical, protective talisman. It has been a favorite for centuries, often grown in the courtyards of monasteries and public gardens. The roots and seeds are both used medicinally and appear in a number of Old World patent medicines. They flavor gin and vermouth, and the liqueurs Chartreuse and Bénédictine. Various local species are sometimes used interchangeably with *A. archangelica.*

Description

Angelica is a stately biennial that attracts immediate attention: It can attain a height of over 6 feet, and its broad, pointed, serrated leaves and stout, hollow, flowering stalks are striking. The small greenish white flowers are arranged in large spherical umbels and develop into plump, pungent seeds.

Preparations and Dosage
Use up to 4.5 grams (0.16 ounces) daily of the chopped root in decoctions, tinctures, and syrups, or soaked in honey. This herb is best used before or around mealtimes. To use the seed, we recommend preparing it as a standard infusion, not as a tincture.

Healing Properties

All parts of angelica, in the form of elixirs, teas, tinctures, and other preparations, are used for enhancing digestion and relieving stomachaches, nausea, and gas pains, as well as symptoms of the common cold. The tender leaves are delightfully tangy and can be chopped up and added to salads, and the tender stems and roots can add a savory taste to soups and other dishes. Candied angelica stems are an old-fashioned treat to "help the medicine go down."

Several Chinese species of angelica, especially *A. dahurica*, are easy to grow and are used as teas for relieving cramps and pain during the menstrual cycle, as well as for their digestive benefits.

Another related species, *A. sinensis*, is the famous Chinese herb dang quai (or dong gui), which is arguably the world's most widely used herb. It is indicated particularly for health problems specific to women: it increases energy, regulates the menstrual cycle, and alleviates pain.

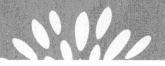

Safety

Some minor safety concerns include an increase in sun sensitivity, allergies, and a possible interaction with anticoagulant therapy. These apply only to the tincture, as heating in a tea or while cooking and drying the root before use reduce these concerns. However, don't use angelica during pregnancy or if you are on anticoagulant therapy, just to be safe.

In the Garden

In angelica's native northern Europe, it likes to grow close to water and can be found on the fringes of boggy areas. In addition, it prefers cooler climates, so if you're in a warmer region, place this plant in the shade and give it rich, moist, yet well-drained soil. Leave plenty of room for a large, 5- to 8-foot beauty, and remove the flowering stalk (if you can bear it) to redirect the plant's energy to the root and increase its quality. In the cooler fall, start it from seed, which germinates best when it's fresh or refrigerated for 6 to 8 weeks. In temperate regions, it will self-seed readily (especially the seeds from the central umbel of flowers). It flowers in its second year and in temperate climates can become a short-lived perennial. You'll love the way insects buzz around it happily in your garden.

Harvesting Angelica: Dig the root during the dormant period—from late fall through early spring—after one or two seasons of growth. Collect the seeds for medicine when they are turning from green to yellow. Be sure to harvest them soon after ripening, because they can rot after heavy rains or even dew. Cut the root into small slices or pieces and use relatively high heat when drying. And watch for insect infestations in storage—dried angelica is really attractive to critters.

Agastache foeniculum

Family: Lamiaceae

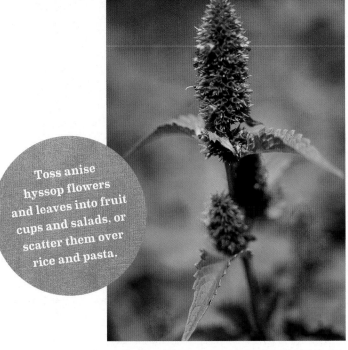

Toss anise hyssop flowers and leaves into fruit cups and salads, or scatter them over rice and pasta.

Anise hyssop

A sweeter herb you could not grow and use! Not only does it taste good enough to snack on directly from the garden, but the soft, sweet-smelling leaves are also lovely to behold and attract bees and butterflies by the dozens. Anise hyssop is native to the north midwestern United States and Canada in open, dry woodlands and prairies, and its close cousin Korean mint (*A. rugosa*) originates in similar regions in Asia.

Description

This erect, columnar perennial grows 2 to 3 feet tall and finishes off with dramatic slender spikes of lavender flowers that appear in midsummer to late summer. The leaves can become tinged with purple in cold weather. Plants usually live for 2 to 3 years before they decline, and they're not fully cold hardy.

Preparations and Dosage

Make a tea with the leaves and young stems. In summer, add ice and lemon for a cooling and digestive beverage. In winter, drink the tea warm throughout the day and before bedtime to help ease into a refreshing sleep. Add the fresh chopped leaves to all kinds of culinary dishes and desserts.

Healing Properties

Anise hyssop adds an inviting aroma and a touch of sweetness to salads, soups, and other dishes. You can top meals with a sprinkling of finely chopped leaves for a unique culinary experience that you might want to use regularly. In addition to the sparkling flavor of anise hyssop and its relatives, the herb also has beneficial health properties, which include preventing and relieving nausea, poor appetite, gas, and abdominal pain. In traditional Chinese medicine, herbalists often recommend drinking anise hyssop as a warm tea throughout a cold or flu to help ease a sore throat and gently reduce a fever.

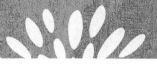

Safety

No safety concerns are known.

In the Garden

These beauties love moist, rich, well-drained soil, and you'll find that full sun with afternoon shade is ideal. They can be sensitive to fungus if kept too wet. Fertilize with liquid seaweed once during the season—it increases leaf size and production. If you have more than mild freezes in your area, grow anise hyssop in a protected area in pots. In mild climates the plants will return after the winter dieback and will even reseed. Starting plants from seed is easy in a greenhouse or a porch window. You can also propagate anise hyssop from cuttings and by root division.

Harvesting Anise Hyssop:
Gather the leaves or aerial parts from early to full flower, including the top fleshy portion of the stem. You'll get multiple harvests in 1 year if you cut the stems just above their first branching to encourage regrowth. Like other members of the mint family, the medicinal potency of anise hyssop is higher later in the growing season, when the weather is quite warm. When drying the plants, bundle them for the hang method, or discard the larger stems and spread them thinly. They'll dry quite quickly.

Cynara scolymus

Family: Asteraceae

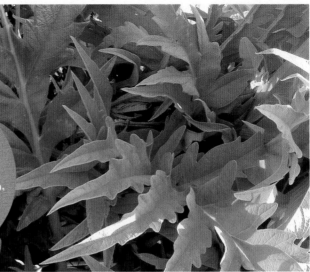

This herb is a "two-fer"— a delicious vegetable and a medicinal herb, all in one plant!

Artichoke

If your only experience with this plant is the delicious vegetable (which is actually its flowerhead), you have no idea what you're missing! Larger than life and very similar in appearance to its cousin cardoon (*C. cardunculus*), artichoke will make a bold statement in your garden with its vivid purple heads, as well as a welcome addition to your medicine cabinet. It's really too bad you can't fit it on your windowsill!

Description

This short-lived perennial can reach a height of 15 feet and a width of 5 feet in one growing season. It is stout and whitish grey, with a sturdy central stalk, large, sharply divided rough leaves, and the familiar head that opens to a purple thistlelike flower.

Preparations and Dosage

Make a standard infusion and drink ½ to 1 cup before meals as desired. Tincturing the leaf is a good way to capture the bitter digestive-enhancing compounds, and since the tincture is easy to carry and has a shelf life of 2 to 3 years, this is a convenient way to use the herb. Follow the label directions for commercial products in capsule and tablet form.

Healing Properties

Pieces of artichoke leaf can be picked and chewed right from the garden. They contain stimulating enzymes that enhance digestion. The taste of the raw leaves is bitter, but most find it enjoyable, which is why it has become popular in elixirs and aperitifs before meals. Why not just eat the artichoke heads? you might ask. Once you taste the leaves, you will realize the difference: The leaves are much stronger-tasting and stronger-acting than the delicious heads.

Artichoke leaf is recommended today to help stimulate your liver and bile, especially when you are having trouble digesting fats. Traditional Chinese medicine speaks of "liver stagnation," which is thought to be a common syndrome that occurs when stress is coupled with a rich diet. Associated symptoms include a headache in the temple area, irritability, and an irregular menstrual cycle. Regular use of artichoke leaf tea or extract can help prevent these unpleasant symptoms.

Recent research has shown that artichoke leaf extract has a mild but significant cholesterol-lowering effect, and it is added to supplements that promote heart health.

Safety

There are no safety concerns in the literature. Theoretical concerns include mild allergic reactions such as digestive upset or a skin rash (but they are usually mild and will go away once you stop consuming the plant), as well as the possibility that artichoke supplements might be a problem for people with bile obstruction or gallbladder disease. Use artichoke under the advice of an experienced herbalist if you have these conditions. Allergic reactions can occur with artichoke.

In the Garden

An artichoke will command a lot of respect in your garden and will be quite easy to grow, as a good vegetable should be (until it gets so tall that it starts to fall over—have supports ready for late summer). You can place it in the back, in a nice, warm spot with well-fertilized soil and consistent water. In mild climates it will return each year, but in four-season climates you'll likely need to seed it each year. Side shoots sometimes form from the base of the plant (though not always in the first year), and you can break them off from the mother plant, pot them up, and take them inside for the winter. Seeds are easy. You can start them in early spring indoors or in late spring directly in the garden.

Harvesting Artichoke: Cut the leaves at the base with scissors or clippers (snipping off the pointed, thorny tips), and slice them into strips for drying.

Withania somnifera

Family: Solanaceae

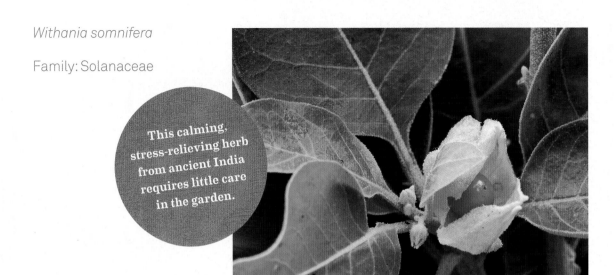

This calming, stress-relieving herb from ancient India requires little care in the garden.

Ashwagandha

In Sanskrit, the word *ashwagandha* means "sweat of the horse," either because of the strong aroma of the root or its reputation for increasing virility. Sometimes called Indian ginseng, it enjoys a revered status in Ayurvedic medicine. Ashwagandha has an astounding ability to address issues that often plague us in our complex, revved-up Western culture.

Description

This tender perennial hails from the hot, dry plains of India and has an appearance not unlike a tomato or potato plant, but with bright green, smooth, oval-shaped leaves. It has a graceful bushy shape and can grow to 3 feet tall and wide. The small green flowers give way to shiny orange-red fruits in a papery casing. The fruits are quite bitter but edible.

Preparations and Dosage

As you'll often find with herbs used in traditional medicine, ashwagandha is usually combined with other tonic herbs, such as ginseng, in commercial formulas, so follow the label recommendations for dosing. To make a decoction of ashwagandha, use 3 to 6 grams of the root each day, and drink ½ to 1 cup of the decoction in the morning and evening. The berries can substitute for rennet in cheese making.

Healing Properties

In India, ashwagandha has been a popular herb for promoting longevity and increasing energy, fertility, and male potency, among many other uses—which sounds a lot like the ways ginseng is used in Chinese culture. Herbal practitioners in many Western countries today recommend root preparations as a tonic for promoting a feeling of "relaxed energy" that simultaneously counteracts the harmful effects of stress. It is often prescribed, along with healthy lifestyle changes, for infertility, impotence, fatigue, insomnia, and arthritis.

Scientific studies show that the root has anti-inflammatory and antioxidant effects, and it supports functional balance of the immune, endocrine, cardiopulmonary, and nervous systems. This defines a true adaptogen, an herb thought to help protect against stress and promote wellness. Other studies show that taking ashwagandha increases urine volume and significantly decreases serum cholesterol, triglycerides, and blood sugar levels.

Even though there are not yet many human studies supporting the traditional uses of ashwagandha, the ones that have been conducted affirm the long historical and traditional uses of the herb.

Safety

No studies have turned up any safety concerns for short-term use, and no clinical reports of side effects or drug interactions have been reported in the medical literature. Traditional use suggests, but doesn't prove, that ashwagandha is generally safe in every case for long-term use. Digestive upset and mild allergic reactions are the most common side effects of taking herbs, especially on an empty stomach, and this is possible while taking ashwagandha, as well.

In the Garden

This tender perennial loves hot, dry weather, so give it full sun and well-drained, average or sandy soil. It will only need water during extreme heat or drought conditions. Expect to treat it as an annual unless you live in a nearly tropical or truly tropical zone—it will probably not survive even a light freeze in the winter. You can give it a big pot and protect it against a south wall, if you like. Propagate it from cuttings or seed, but remember that it needs light and temperatures above 70°F to germinate.

Harvesting Ashwagandha: The root can be harvested after winter dieback or the first frost during the first year (or the second or third year, if you live in a warm enough area to see your ashwagandha return). Roots will rot in cold, wet soil. The aerial parts are sometimes also used medicinally in traditional Ayurvedic medicine, but they're fairly bitter (especially the berries). Harvest when the berries are red and ripe. In Ayurveda, the root is nearly always boiled in milk prior to drying. Whether you follow this process or not, cut the root into small, uniform pieces to dry it.

Astragalus membranaceus

Family: Fabaceae

A powerful immunity herb, astragalus is used in formulas to prevent serious illness.

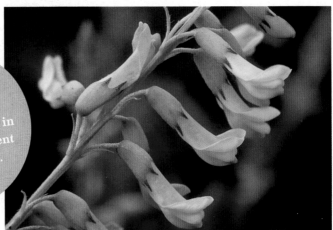

Astragalus

Two thousand years ago in China, astragalus (or huang qi) was listed in *Shen Nong's Herbal* as a tonic, and indeed, it is the quintessential herb for immunity. Ginseng and Astragalus Combination (Bu Zhong Yi Qi Tang) tonic, created during the Yuan Dynasty in the 13th century, is still used today to increase strength and endurance. Although astragalus root arose in China as a cultural treasure, it has made its way into Western healing systems worldwide as a "superior herb" for "restoring the normal," which means that with regular use it helps to correct the underlying conditions that can lead to illnesses like cancer and chronic fatigue.

Description

Astragalus often has a sprawling habit unless it is staked, but it can become upright as it ages. The plant looks very much like the pea family–member that it is, with the typical pinnately compound leaves and yellow blossoms that mature into pealike seedpods. It can reach 3 to 5 feet in height.

Preparations and Dosage

Add astragalus root to soups and other dishes to make a strengthening tonic, as they do in Chinese culture. You'll find preparations of the root in natural food stores and herb shops (dried root slices are available in bulk) to make decoctions, as well as extracts, tablets, and capsules.

Take 9 to 15 grams of dried and prepared, sliced or shredded root. You can simmer 4 or 5 medium astragalus slices in 4 cups of water, along with other tonic herbs (like licorice), and drink 1 cup in the morning and 1 cup in the evening. Follow the label directions on commercial products.

Healing Properties

Compounds from the roots have been shown to slow the aging process in animal cells by helping to preserve the length of telomeres at the ends of chromosomes. Long telomere length has been associated with human longevity, which might explain the reverence with which this herb is held in traditional Chinese culture.

Astragalus promotes the production of white blood cells, helping your body produce antibodies and interferon to fight infections. Herbalists often recommend it for times when you experience frequent colds and flu, fatigue, and weakness in your limbs (when your arms and legs feel heavy). With regular use, astragalus is thought to be one of the most important herbs to help strengthen your immune system and to help your body prevent and fight cancer and chronic viral syndromes. It is especially indicated for use during recovery from a serious or long illness because it promotes strong digestion and assimilation of nutrients. In the case of chronic illness, the herb is often taken daily for anywhere from 3 months to several years or more. More well-designed modern human trials are needed to confirm its status as a major healing herb for mainstream medical practice, but even without them, astragalus continues to be used widely in many cultures.

Safety

Safety concerns are minimal, and there are no contraindications during pregnancy. But keep in mind that in traditional Chinese medicine, tonic herbs are thought to strengthen the pathogen along with the immune system, and so are sometimes avoided during fevers in the acute phase of an infection.

In the Garden

Astragalus grows along the margins of forests and grasslands in dry, sandy soil in its native Mongolia and northeastern China, so do your best to give it the same conditions: full sun and deep, sandy, well-drained soil. (Poor drainage will cause the root to rot in winter.) Cultivate the soil deeply. This perennial is moderately drought tolerant and doesn't need to be fertilized, but it is prone to gophers, so provide netting to protect it. The seed needs to be stratified, scarified, or soaked overnight in an inoculant. Astragalus is one of the first things you can start in the cold soil of your early spring greenhouse or on your back porch, with very reliable germination—or start it outside in the fall for spring germination. It can tolerate high heat and a winter freeze.

Harvesting Astragalus: The root is collected after the fourth or fifth year of growth, in autumn, after the plant has died back. Use a digging fork, as astragalus has a long taproot. Slice it lengthwise or cut it into small, uniform pieces for drying.

Ocimum basilicum and
O. tenuiflorum, syn. *O. sanctum*

Family: Lamiaceae

Rub the leaves of tulsi on your skin to soothe itchy insect bites.

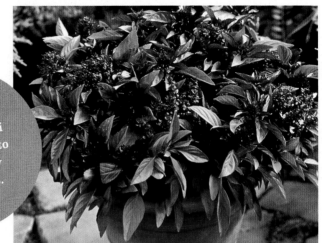

Basil *and* Tulsi

The many varieties of culinary basil are well known and loved for their savory contributions to modern dishes, but that's nothing compared to Greek and Roman times, when basil could only be grown by those of noble blood. In India, its close relative, tulsi (also known as holy basil)—sacred to the god Vishnu's wife, Lakshmi—is grown outside every home for good fortune and is known as a virtual panacea.

Description

Most of us recognize our common culinary basil, which has large, tender, ovate leaves and succulent stems, as an annual commonly found in the vegetable patch. Tulsi is similar, but it's upright and branching, and usually smaller and sturdier in all but the warmest climates. The green or purplish leaves are often smaller and the stems are quite stiff (the base can even become woody), and they can have a purplish tinge, as well. In hot areas like those in tulsi's native India, the plant can reach 2 feet tall. The bluish purple flowers keep coming as fast as you can remove them!

Preparations and Dosage

We probably don't need to tell you to liberally add basil to your culinary dishes or to put up lots of pesto while basil is in season! You can also make a nice tea with culinary basil, or infuse basil in oil to use for treating skin conditions. It makes a lovely bath herb that is quite fragrant and soothing. Tulsi makes a pungent and alluring tea, tincture, oil, and salve, and it is found commercially in extract form. The recommended dosage is 2 capsules, twice daily.

Healing Properties

Culinary basil is considered a delightful digestive aid and nervine (an herb that affects the nervous system). In some European countries, it is used externally as an antifungal for conditions such as athlete's foot, and also as an insect repellent. In South America, it is used for respiratory and rheumatic problems and to allay nausea and pain.

Tulsi is widely used in Ayurvedic medicine as a longevity tonic, as an adaptogen to help alleviate stress and tension, and to treat upper respiratory conditions such as bronchitis. Studies show that it has potent antibacterial, antifungal, immunomodulatory, and anti-inflammatory effects, and that it reduces blood glucose levels in diabetics. Herbalists recommend it for generalized anxiety disorders, and studies support this use. It has also been studied and recommended for its ability to safely preserve foods.

Tulsi contains within its volatile oil the substance eugenol, which has been widely studied for its anti-inflammatory properties. Many holistic practitioners and medical researchers believe that most, if not all, chronic disease results from chronic inflammation, making tulsi one of the best herbs you can take for your overall health and longevity.

Safety

Basil and tulsi are both widely and regularly used as spices around the world, which would support the idea that they are safe to use as healing herbs, as well. Some concerns about interaction with blood thinners and other medications have been voiced, but they are theoretical only. As teas or when used in cooking, both types of basil are safe. Use caution during pregnancy other than occasional use in cooking.

In the Garden

Both types of basil need warmth and full sun, average to rich soil with plenty of humus, and regular irrigation. Fertilize them well if you are planting in the same spot year after year. Tulsi is frost sensitive, but hardier and more drought tolerant than culinary basil. It will self-seed and even die back in autumn and return the following summer in warm areas. Culinary basil is always grown as an annual, except in the tropics. Pinch back the flowering stalk of either plant to prolong leaf growth and stimulate bushiness. (This will also prevent tulsi from crossbreeding if several varieties are being grown together.) Fungal diseases can take hold if the plants don't have good air circulation. Start from seed in a warm greenhouse or sunny window, or direct-sow in the garden after the soil has warmed, just pressing the seed into the soil but not covering it.

Harvesting Culinary Basil and Tulsi: Gather the leaves and stems, pinching the plant back often, and include the flower in your tea or medicine preparation. Keep both basils cool as you are harvesting, as they hold heat and blacken easily. Remove any thick stems before drying, and remember that the leaves dry quickly. Make sure that the drying heat is not set too high, and take extra care to dry basil in darkness, as it easily browns or blackens when exposed to sunlight. Both varieties are excellent candidates for freezing.

Arctium lappa

Family: Asteraceae

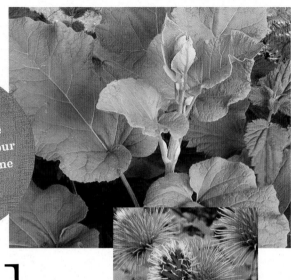

Burdock strengthens the vital energy of your body and immune system.

Burdock

If you live in the eastern part of the country, you probably know this "weed," even though you think you don't. It's considered invasive in many regions of the United States and grows spontaneously in many parts of the world, especially in places with summer rain. The root is sold in Asian markets and in supermarket produce departments as "gobo," and it and the leaves have been staples of the cuisine for thousands of years. In 1948, when the Swiss inventor George de Mestral observed the action of the burrs on his dog's fur, the inspiration for Velcro was born!

Description

Burdock is a bold, stout biennial that sports large, coarse, heart-shaped leaves in its first year and a tiered group of flowering stalks with purple thistlelike flowers that mature to burrs in its second year. And with some varieties, grown in the right conditions, you may even see flowers and burrs the first year. It can range from 1 foot high and slender to more than 8 feet tall and several feet wide.

Preparations and Dosage
Burdock root can be prepared as a decoction, tincture, or dried extract. Take ½ to 1 teaspoon of the tincture in a little water several times a day. Make a decoction with 10 to 30 grams of the dried root and drink 1 or 2 cups a day before or with meals. Capsules or tablets containing burdock root extract should be taken as directed.

Healing Properties

The root and seed are used for their strengthening actions on the immune and digestive systems. Burdock is a great example of a class of herbs called alteratives, which are thought to help your body maintain homeostasis (a stable and healthy internal environment). This likely helps to maintain blood sugar and immune balance. Japanese cuisine makes regular use of burdock, often featuring it in a dish called *kinpira gobo*. As part of a regular diet, the root is thought to promote strength and vitality, making it a *qi* tonic. ("Qi" means "vital energy" in traditional Chinese medicine and culture.)

Burdock is known in Western herbalism as both an alterative and an immune system booster, and it is widely used in teas and extracts for relieving liver congestion and difficulty digesting fats. The root and seed are also recommended for rheumatism and arthritis, gout, and as a cancer preventive. (Research has shown that burdock root demonstrates anticancer properties.) The seed is used in traditional Chinese herbal practice to heal skin ailments such as acne, boils, and eczema.

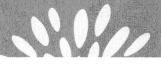

Safety

Burdock is known to be safe for use without restriction and for all ages. There are no contraindications for use during pregnancy.

In the Garden

Burdock will adapt to almost any soil or growing condition, although it prefers alkaline soil and full sun. It volunteers in open places and disturbed soil, and it doesn't need fertilizer, but it does rely on regular moisture. Start it from seed. (Direct sowing is easy. You can help the process along by breaking up the mature, dry seedheads in autumn and scattering the contents.) Burdock seed likes to go through a cold winter, or you can stratify the seeds, but they won't germinate until the soil is warm.

Harvesting Burdock: Dig the root in the fall of the first year, after the plant has died back, or in the spring of the second year, before the flowering stalk has emerged. When collecting the seed, remember that it has accompanying small hairs that can be irritating to your skin, so wear gloves, long sleeves, and even eye protection if you have a large amount to harvest. Break open the dried seedheads to separate out the seed, or use a seed cleaner. Cut the root into small, uniform pieces for drying. It needs relatively high heat to dry thoroughly. Keep the seed in a paper bag in a dry place and shake the bag every so often to disperse any moisture. After a week, store the seed properly.

Calendula officinalis

Family: Asteraceae

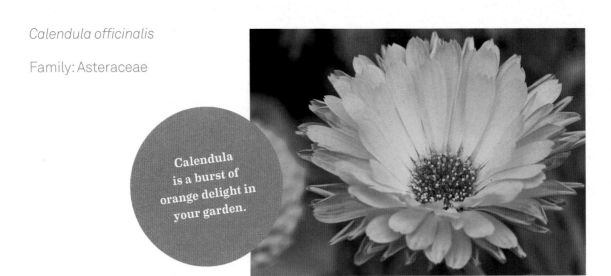

Calendula is a burst of orange delight in your garden.

Calendula

Whether displaying bright orange or sunny yellow flowers, calendula (also called pot marigold) is one of the most essential parts of your garden medicine chest: Those aromatic flowering heads can be collected and made into oils and salves to help heal skin injuries of all kinds. Make sure you grow only *C. officinalis,* and not any of the many "marigolds" (*Tagetes* spp.) or selected ornamental varieties that are available. Once you get it going, it will return every season to light up your garden.

Description

This beautiful annual, which often self-seeds from year to year, has orange or yellow daisylike flowers at various points along its green, fleshy, branching stem. It blooms from summer until winter's freezing temperatures (and even year-round, in its native, hot areas of Africa). The plant can grow to almost 2 feet tall, and the flowers tend to open with sunny, dry weather and close in low temperatures or when there's impending rain.

Preparations and Dosage

Use the freshly dried flower-heads to make creams, salves, liniments, teas, tinctures, and oils, or add the flowerheads directly to your bath to soothe irritated skin. For internal conditions, take 1 to 3 droppersful of tincture in a little water several times daily. Sprinkle the fresh flower petals onto salads, spreads, and other dishes to add a dash of vivid natural color!

Healing Properties

Use the entire flowerhead (not just the petals) in preparations for healing cuts, scrapes, burns, sunburn, diaper rash, sores, ulcers, varicose veins, chapped dry skin and lips, and insect bites. Salves, oils, creams, and other preparations can be found in drug stores and natural food stores alike, since calendula has long been the go-to herb for these skin problems. Science shows that extracts of the flowerheads have anti-inflammatory and antibacterial effects. And herbalists have long recommended tea infusions of calendula to help heal ulcers in the digestive tract, soothe gallbladder inflammation, and treat enlarged, sore lymph glands. Research has uncovered an antiherpes virus action, as well, and the cream is often applied to ease the pain and inflammation of herpes sores.

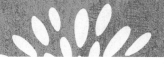

Safety

As with other members of the daisy family, some people are sensitive to calendula because of the sesquiterpene compounds that the plant contains. If you have allergic skin reactions or are unusually sensitive to foods or the environment, start with a low dose of this herb and work up to a full dose, if you don't experience any reaction.

In the Garden

This lovely, sunny flower enjoys full sun—or even partial shade, in hot-summer regions—and average soil, and has moderate water needs. If flower production dwindles, you can cut back the plants, even drastically, to increase new flower production. Calendula will self-sow yearly in many gardens, and it doesn't mind crowding. Direct-sow the seed in early spring or late fall, as it can withstand some frost; with a little luck, you'll have it always!

Harvesting Calendula: Collect the flowerheads on hot, sunny days for the highest resin content, and pick them regularly to prevent the plants from putting their energy into seed production. Once that happens, the rest of the flowers will be smaller. Choose flowers that are just opening in the morning before 11 a.m. Dry calendula quickly after you harvest it, and be sure to check the center of the flower for dryness. Molding in storage is a common problem! Watch for reabsorption of moisture, and keep it in complete darkness, since the flowers fade easily.

Eschscholzia californica

Family: Papaveraceae

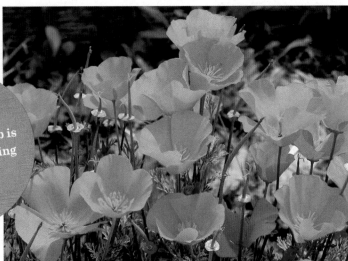

> Called "cup of gold" by the Spanish, this herb is powerfully calming and safe for all ages.

California poppy

The state flower of California is a wondrous sight to behold in the spring, when vast hillsides and fields light up with its vibrant color. Sometimes considered to be the "gold" in the Golden State, this wild, low-growing beauty will make a great addition to your garden, often reseeding to bring both beauty and healing year after year.

Description

The attractive grayish green and reddish feathery leaves of California poppy are topped by golden, cup-shaped flowers on long stalks that last until the first killing frost. Slender, spear-shaped seedpods follow as the plant blooms on. The bright orange, translucent roots contain up to three times the active compounds found in the foliage, but all parts of this plant are used medicinally.

Preparations and Dosage

The whole plant is often used, though the root is the strongest part. Take 2 to 4 droppersful or 1 teaspoon of the tincture in a little water or herb tea as needed, up to three or four times daily. Use 1 to 4 droppersful at night to remedy sleeplessness in children. The tea is rather bitter, but infusions can be made with 1 cup of boiling water poured over 1 to 2 teaspoons of dried herb and infused for 10 minutes. Follow the label directions on commercial products.

The edible flowers can be used to beautifully decorate salads, casseroles, and desserts for a summer feast.

Healing Properties

California poppy tea was used by American Indians to help soothe fussy babies and to promote a calm and healing sleep for their parents. The root contains a variety of nonnarcotic alkaloids that have been shown to relax smooth muscle, especially in the uterus and bronchial airways, treating menstrual cramps and spasmodic coughs.

Poppy teas, tinctures, and other preparations are recommended by herbalists for relieving anxiety, nervousness, stomach and uterine cramps, and bronchial constriction. California poppy promotes healthy sleep and is a mild pain reliever. Health professionals use it to help their patients slowly reduce prescription drug use and withdraw from addictive substances, as well as to treat children with hyperactive tendencies.

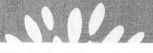

Safety

Safety concerns are all theoretical. For instance, the extract, because it is mildly sedative, has been suggested to strengthen the effects of pharmaceutical sedatives—but that's very unlikely to happen in practice. A clinical study that followed 264 participants for 3 months showed that California poppy plus hawthorn and magnesium was just as safe as—and more effective than—a placebo treatment for reducing mild to moderate anxiety. The safety of California poppy during pregnancy has not been studied, but no harmful effects have been noted.

In the Garden

This California native likes warm, dry, sandy soil and full sun. You can lightly water it during periods of active growth, but it does best if you give it dry conditions while it's flowering. Don't overfertilize. In warm climates, if it looks spent after flowering, you can renew it by cutting it back to the ground and watering it a bit. Start it from seed (stratification helps), and direct-sow it in fall or early spring, since it rarely transplants well. You might find that it self-sows and spreads very easily in warm, dry climates. When grouping California poppies with other flowers, give the poppies 12 to 16 inches all around— they really extend.

Harvesting California Poppy:

Collect the aerial parts or the whole plant while the flowers are still blooming and the seedpods are present. Dig the root after fall dieback. Dry it and the aerial parts separately, so you don't overdry the thinner portions. All parts of the plant, particularly the aboveground portions, are easily degraded by sunlight. California poppy is delicate in storage, but it will last 18 months if kept in an airtight container.

Nepeta cataria

Family: Lamiaceae

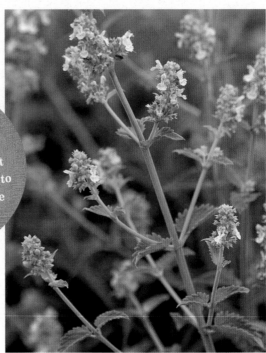

Rub catnip on your skin to repel insects, or finely mince it and add it to culinary sauces to add an undertone of mint.

Catnip

Who doesn't know about catnip's reputation? It turns out that only about two-thirds of all cats react with delirium to this plant and that there are many factors involved. But the compound in catnip that attracts tabbies (nepetalactone) is also responsible for an insecticidal action. You'll find catnip in many deet-free sprays. If you want to protect your plant from marauding felines, place a wire basket upside down over it—and weight it down.

Description

This short-lived branching perennial grows up to 3 feet high with a somewhat rangy profile. It has feltlike, gray-green, heart-shaped leaves; small white flowers; stiff stems; and a strong aroma. You might find that it self-seeds in sunny, disturbed soil like ditches and pastures. It doesn't mind a winter freeze, yet it can also handle high heat.

Preparations and Dosage

Catnip can be stuffed into toy mice for your feline friends to enjoy, and bathing or sponging your pets with catnip tea (when they'll comply) can help discourage fleas. For children, make up to a quart of the strong infusion, and administer it throughout the day for a few days or up to 1 week to treat fevers associated with infections. You can also add 1 teaspoon of tincture to 2 cups of water, or to a peppermint infusion, and drink it ½ cup at a time throughout the day.

Healing Properties

Catnip makes a rather pleasant tea infusion, especially with a little sweetener added, for children who are fussy and colicky. It can also help to lower a child's fever and calm his or her discomfort. Since fevers are an important part of a child's immune response, it's good to start with a catnip infusion before resorting to stronger medications. Give young children (under 5 years old) teaspoons of a catnip and honey infusion throughout the day, and if the fever spikes, try giving the child a short cool bath or cool catnip tea compresses along with the tea taken internally. We recommend blending catnip with lemon balm and any of the mints—peppermint or spearmint—to increase potency and improve the flavor.

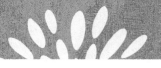

Safety

Catnip has no known safety concerns and is considered safe for children. Some authorities have contraindicated it during pregnancy because of its traditional use to regulate the menstrual flow, though no evidence is available to support this concern.

In the Garden

With the exception of very mucky ground, catnip grows well in all soil types, including dry, sandy, and gravelly. Give it full sun or partial shade, and keep it dry to increase the volatile oil production in the aromatic leaf. Cut it back to the ground, or at least back by half, at each harvest, and a second growth will come quickly. The plant itself will be short-lived, but will probably self-sow in the garden. You can propagate it from seed (it needs warm soil and light to germinate), from cuttings, or by root division. It is prone to thrips and white fly infestations, which spot the leaves but don't affect their medicinal value.

Harvesting Catnip: Collect healthy, nonyellowing leaves and tops when the plant is in flower. The leaves can bruise if you're not gentle when separating them from the stem. The second-year harvest is the best one, and the medicine is strongest when some of the flowers are past their prime and are browning. If you're sensitive, wear gloves and even a dust mask when you'll be harvesting a lot of this herb: It's a strong sedative and can leave a metallic taste in your mouth after prolonged skin exposure. When drying, take only the leaves—don't include any stem—and you'll find that it dries quickly.

Capsicum annuum

Family: Solanaceae

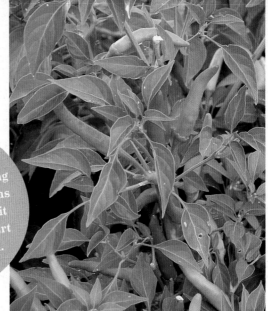

This herb is hot! It's in pain-relieving prescription creams for shingles, and it benefits your heart and circulation.

Cayenne

Talk about popular herbs—this one is *hot*. Cayenne peppers were carried back to Europe from Columbus's travels to the New World. Its primary constituent, capsaicin, is the active ingredient in personal protection sprays and animal repellents. Numerous varieties of *Capsicum* have been developed or selected: Some peppers are fiery hot, like Thai chiles, and some are quite mild, like the bell pepper. Paprika spice is derived from a related species, and *C. frutescens* is the source material for Tabasco sauce.

Description

This spicy fruit is a perennial shrub in its native South America, but it's usually grown as an annual in northern gardens. It resembles other members of its family, such as bell peppers, and is dense and compact, with smaller, glossy, lance-shaped leaves. It can grow to a height of about 2 feet, and its small, star-shaped white flowers are followed by green pods (fruits) that ripen to red or yellow.

Preparations and Dosage

Use cayenne in capsules, tablets, or tinctures, and sprinkle it on your food.

Take 1 to 4 capsules of the powder twice daily. For the tincture, use 1 to 4 droppersful two or three times a day. Or make an infusion by pouring 1 cup of boiling water over 1 teaspoon of freshly crushed dried seeds or fruits and letting it steep for 10 to 15 minutes before straining out the herb. Add honey and lemon juice, then drink as needed.

Healing Properties

Cayenne is an important circulatory herb, and it was enthusiastically recommended by herbalists of the early 20th century, especially the famed Dr. John Christopher, for just about any ailment. His son, David, told us that his dad would often amaze members of the audience by consuming large quantities with nary a whimper—even placing it in his eyes. He recommended cayenne to improve digestion; reduce cholesterol; benefit the heart, blood, and blood vessels; and reduce various pains in the body, such as joint pain, digestive pain, nerve pain, and headaches. He also recommended applying it to the skin to treat shingles, neuralgias, and arthritis. Today, preparations of cayenne's main constituent, capsaicin, are found in prescription medications for treating the pain of shingles and sore joints.

Capsaicin can produce an intense burning sensation when it touches your skin, but this subsides with continued use. Applications of cayenne to your skin can stimulate endorphins and block pain-signaling chemicals, inducing a feeling of well-being and sometimes even euphoria. Why do you think hot chiles are so popular in some cultures? It's all about the high!

Safety

Avoid getting cayenne in your eyes. (Yes, it is used medicinally for cataracts, but don't try it at home!) The active components transfer easily to your hands, mouth, genitalia, and other mucous membranes, so wear gloves when handling the peppers and wash your hands thoroughly afterward. The heat from the fruit is actually concentrated in the white fluffy partitions (called the placenta), not in the seeds, as is often assumed.

In the Garden

This popular spicy fruit needs full sun, hot weather, and a long growing season to thrive. It requires a moderate amount of water and rich soil. Start the seeds in a spring greenhouse and keep them on a sunny windowsill or patio. (Scarifying the seeds or soaking them in gibberellic acid will aid germination.) Keep them inside and in the sun or plant out when the weather warms up, and then make sure you harden them off for outdoor growth before transplanting. (Acclimate them by setting them outside for longer and longer periods with each passing day.) Space the plants in your garden at 1- to 2-foot intervals, and stake them if they begin to droop as they grow. Mulch well.

Harvesting Cayenne: Collect cayenne fruits by cutting, not pulling, them from the plants, and be sure to wear gloves. Red peppers are traditionally dried in the sun on sloped boards or on hillsides. You can dry them whole in the dehydrator or oven, set to the lowest temperature setting, or gather them together by their stems and hang them to dry from a rafter in a warm kitchen.

Matricaria recutita and
Chamaemelum nobile,
syn. *Anthemis nobilis*

Family: Asteraceae

In Mexico and South America, this herb is grown outside the door for good health.

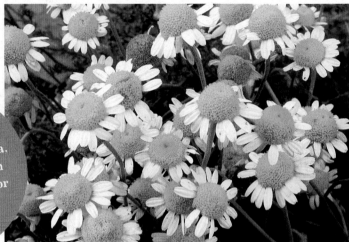

Chamomile

Peter Rabbit's mother was right: This charming flower soothes a troubled tummy and calms a restless child. Most chamomile that you find commercially will be the German (*M. recutita*), which is much preferred to and better studied than the Roman (*C. nobile,* syn. *A. nobilis*), and it's definitely better tasting. The two species can be used in a similar manner, although the Roman is more bitter and less soothing than you'd expect a chamomile to be. It is often found in commercial cosmetic products.

Description

German and Roman chamomiles can be used in similar ways, and they can be mistaken for one another in the garden. German chamomile can grow anywhere from 6 to 24 inches tall and has feathery leaves; small, abundant, daisylike flowers; and a pleasant scent. The Roman looks very much the same, though it's shorter and is often described as a perennial. However, the annual German can perennialize in warm climates.

Preparations and Dosage

German chamomile makes such a pleasant-tasting tea that this has become the standard preparation. Tinctures and extracts in capsules and tablets are also popular.

The key to success with chamomile is to use the freshest herb possible, whether in its fresh or dried form—and nothing is fresher than growing your own! Make up 1 quart of the infusion at a time by adding freshly boiled water to 2 to 4 ounces of the dried flowering tops. Drink 1 cup at a time, three to five times daily. If you're using the tincture, add ½ to 1 teaspoon of it to a cup of warm water.

Healing Properties

The chamomiles are especially revered for easing digestive woes, and *manzanilla*, as German chamomile is known in Spanish, is known by most every Latin American parent for the calming and comforting effect it can have on children. The tea is recommended by herbalists for easing intestinal cramps and irritation, indigestion, ulcers, and colic, as well as nervousness, insomnia, fever, and teething in children. It also soothes muscle cramps, aches and pains of flu, headaches, neuralgia, and motion sickness. Externally, chamomile tea is used as an eyewash for conjunctivitis and is included in commercial and homemade creams for skin inflammation, burns, and bites.

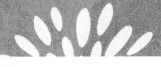

Safety

Allergic reactions to chamomile pollen are rare, and most practitioners consider the herb safe for use by young children and pregnant women.

In the Garden

Chamomile likes moist, light, and sandy loam with good drainage, and it enjoys being crowded. Start it from seed early in the spring so that your harvest will come along before any intense seasonal heat, which tends to stunt flower production. Press the seed into the soil surface, and keep it moist. You can direct-seed into a pot or the ground outdoors, in full sun to partial shade. Keep the growing plants well watered to avoid spindly growth and a low bloom rate. Harvest regularly, or flower production will slow or stop. As the plants get long and straggly and flower production slows, you can mow or cut them back severely, lightly fertilize, and wait for a new flush of flowers. They are frost-hardy.

Harvesting Chamomile: Start harvesting the flowers early in the day, when temperatures are cool. If you have to harvest in the heat, remember that the flowers heat up quickly when piled, and keep them in the shade. You can use a blueberry or chamomile rake, if you have one. Make sure you harvest often: At the beginning of the season, gather flowers every 7 to 10 days, and at summer's peak, do it several times a week. Dry them immediately after harvest, since they degrade quickly.

Symphytum officinale

Family: Boraginaceae

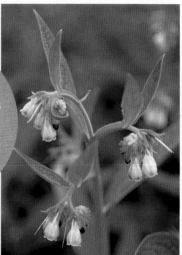

Comfrey is the source of allantoin, a common ingredient in over-the-counter medications for wound healing.

Comfrey

One of comfrey's common names is "knitbone," which refers to its ability to heal broken limbs. It was used by the famous Greek physician Dioscorides as a wound healer in the 1st century, and the word comfrey derives from a Roman term meaning "join together." Despite much past publicity and controversy, comfrey is perfectly safe to use if you follow the proper guidelines. In addition, make sure that you don't substitute a look-alike ornamental hybrid, Russian comfrey (*S. uplandicum*), which has very high levels of toxic alkaloids.

Description

Comfrey is a vigorous, hardy perennial with large, lance-shaped, roughly hairy leaves and pink to purple bell-shaped flowers in drooping clusters on an arching stalk in summer. The root is fleshy and branched, black on the outside and white inside, and is highly mucilaginous. (So are the leaves, when split at the stem.) It grows quickly and spreads easily, even from tiny discarded pieces of the root, which causes growers to exclaim in delight (or moan in despair), "Once you have comfrey, you'll always have comfrey!"

Preparations and Dosage

You can crush and blend comfrey root or leaf with a little water to make a slimy paste and apply it as a poultice, adding more as it dries out. Apply it to external injuries for as long as needed on unbroken skin, and on broken skin, apply it *around* the wound, under the advice of an herbalist.

Comfrey is one of the most popular ingredients in herbal salves and creams, and it makes an effective tincture and tea. The root contains abundant mucilage, which is water soluble but not oil soluble. The other important compound, allantoin, which is a wound-healing substance occurring in high concentrations in the root, and in lesser amounts in the leaves, is at a high concentration only in the juice, root pulp, or powder.

Healing Properties

Comfrey has long been recommended as an external preparation for helping to heal all manner of trauma to the skin and bones. It is used to heal burns, bites, stings, cuts, strains, sprains, and broken bones—taken both internally and externally. Comfrey is also taken internally for lung, bowel, and urinary tract conditions.

Safety

Today, comfrey is most often recommended for external use because it contains toxic alkaloids that have been linked to liver inflammation and toxicity in connection with its internal use. These pyrrolizidine alkaloids, or PAs, are only mildly toxic, but other species are known to have various levels of PAs of high toxicity. (In *S. officinalis*, the young leaves and roots contain the highest levels of PAs.) One reason why commercial products containing comfrey have been discontinued by most manufacturers is the difficulty in determining the species identity when the herb has been powdered or extracted and added to capsules or tablets.

Avoid comfrey if you're pregnant or nursing. Don't use leaf preparations internally for longer than 1 week, twice a year, and always do so under the care of a qualified herbalist. We don't advise using it internally or on broken skin.

Allantoin, however, is a safe and effective cell proliferator. Don't apply it unless a broken bone has been set properly, and don't apply it to a deep, open wound that may not have been cleaned, since it could close at the top before the underlying tissue has fully healed.

In the Garden

Comfrey is native to moist, marshy areas of northern Europe, and indeed, it does thrive and expand rapidly when it's given plenty of water. It likes rich soil, although it's not picky and will be happy in any sunny or shady position in your garden or in a container on your deck. Comfrey tolerates crowding and is so adaptable that virtually nothing but extremely dry conditions will stop its happy rambling. For this reason, it's a great candidate for a pot, indoors or out. Seed is hard to germinate and very erratic, but root division is super easy, even with very small slices.

Harvesting Comfrey: The leaves are optimal when the plant is in early flower. You can continually cut it to the ground and it will rebound quickly with a new set of leaves. Wear gloves if you might be sensitive to the irritating hairs. Dig the root after the plant has died back in the fall and before it reemerges in the spring. It's difficult to get all of the root, so expect comfrey to regrow even when you believe you've completely cleared it! When you're drying the leaves, make sure you turn them often, because they tend to mat together and blacken easily. The root dries slowly because of the dense mucilage. Cut the roots into small, uniform pieces and use the oven method for quicker results.

Echinacea purpurea,
E. angustifolia

Family: Asteraceae

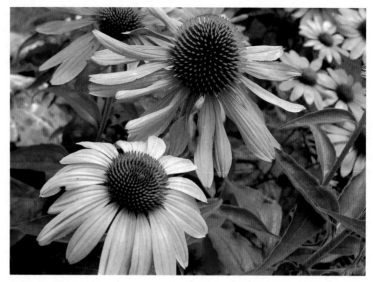

Echinacea

The fantastic popularity echinacea enjoyed during the early 1990s resulted in many fortunes made in the herb industry, and it also resulted in extensive overharvesting of this plant. The root, flowers, and leaves of this North American native were introduced to white settlers by the American Indians (it was an important snake-bite remedy) and rapidly caught the attention of early 20th-century physicians. Although slightly different in their medicinal constituent profiles, both species discussed here are used interchangeably and have become widely used as immune stimulants to fight off common colds and flu. Because overharvesting has endangered wild stands of these plants in many areas, we recommend growing echinacea and contributing to our national heritage of self-care and that of preserving and protecting wild populations. Cultivated echinacea can be just as potent as wild-harvested echinacea and more consistent in its activity. Unlike wild populations, cultivated plants have much less genetic and chemical variation.

This is the world's most famous immune tonic, used to prevent and treat colds and infections.

Description

This beautiful perennial, found commonly in flower gardens and landscape displays, grows 2 to 4 feet tall and sports lovely, large, purple-petaled flowers with cone-shaped, spiny seed-heads that rise above the foliage like lollipops. The rough, dark green, pointed leaves are narrow in the case of *E. angustifolia* and wider in *E. purpurea*. Many new colors of flowering heads are available today—yellow, orange, red, white—so you can find one to fit in with any garden color scheme. However, these color variants have not been tested for their medicinal value.

Safety

There are no known side effects, but use echinacea cautiously and only under the advice of an herbal practitioner if you have an auto-immune condition like lupus or an immune-compromised condition like AIDS or HIV.

Theoretical side effects are sometimes mentioned for echinacea, such as interactions with immunosuppressant therapy. Conservative authors might contraindicate echinacea during pregnancy and nursing, though many herbalists do not. A famous study performed with 206 pregnant women using echinacea during the first trimester showed no observable problems. The authors stated that echinacea should be safe during pregnancy.

Echinacea, like many members of the aster or daisy family, has been occasionally associated with mild allergic reactions. We concur that echinacea should not be used continuously, but mainly when needed, for a few weeks at a time. Why stimulate the immune system all the time? It makes sense that the immune system will stop responding when continuously prodded.

In the Garden

Echinacea originated in the plains, open meadows, sunny woodlands, and prairies of the United States, with *E. angustifolia* having a generally more northern range than *E. purpurea*. Both like full sun or partial shade, but *E. purpurea* requires more water, though not constant moisture. Both plants are frost hardy and can tolerate poor, rocky soils. Try bunching a group of plants for a dramatic effect, or plant one of the dwarf varieties in a pot. Start it from seed, stratifying it or seeding in the fall, if you typically have snowy winters. *Purpurea* is easier to grow (although both take several weeks to germinate) and can also be propagated by root division. You can divide the crown as well, making sure that there are several buds on each section that you replant.

Harvesting Echinacea: The leaves can be harvested starting in the spring, when they're sizing up. The flowers can be harvested when they start to open, but for maximum medicinal potency, harvest the cone when it is mounding. Dig the root in the fall of the third or fourth year, after the plant has died back. Dry the flower by splitting the seedhead, and chop the root into small, uniform pieces before drying.

Echinacea *(Continued from page 32)*

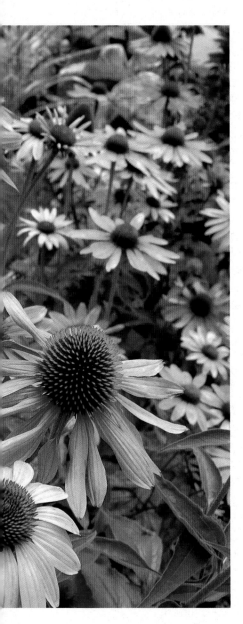

Preparations and Dosage

Tincture preparations of echinacea have been most favored by herbalists, and that's what you'll find most commonly available. In part, this is due to convenience: Echinacea should be taken frequently and regularly to treat symptoms or when trying to ward off an upper respiratory tract infection, and a tincture can go everywhere with you. But the other reason for the prevalence of tinctures is that herbalists feel that echinacea should be extracted fresh and not dried. This is because the most potent active compounds are likely to be fairly unstable after drying, especially when the dried root, flowers, or leaves are powdered or shredded. The active compounds are more stable in an alcoholic solution, and tinctures have a shelf life of at least 2 to 3 years, if they're not left in the sun to overheat.

Take 2 droppersful to 1 teaspoon of tincture three or four times daily, in cycles of 2 weeks on and 1 week off during cold and flu season, or whenever you are feeling run-down and people around you are sick. Label instructions on echinacea tinctures are usually very conservative and should be considered to be on the low side of an effective dose during an active infection.

Make a tea from the fresh (or recently dried) chopped root, flowers, and/or leaves and drink 1 cup two to five times daily. The best tinctures are made from all three plant parts as well, often harvested at different times of year, tinctured separately, and blended later. Follow the label instructions for commercial products.

Healing Properties

The immune-stimulating activity of echinacea, with its main use as a cure for colds, is well known, having been studied and proven repeatedly. Think of the market for a natural remedy that can help reduce the symptoms and duration of a cold with no side effects, derived from a native flower that can easily be grown at home. Why, in the United States alone, it has been estimated that we suffer from about 1 billion colds each year!

The recent popularity of echinacea arose because it does what no pharmaceutical drug can yet do: help reduce the severity and duration of the unpleasant symptoms of colds and flu, allowing us to continue with the activities of our daily lives. Its buzzy taste adds to its mystique, and for some folks, the stronger the better! *E. angustifolia*'s root and the seeds of both species provide the strongest tingle on the tongue, but *E. purpurea* seeds, blended with the roots and leaves of the plant, have been a standard preparation from many commercial manufacturers.

How well does echinacea work to reduce the severity and duration of a cold? Many hundreds of studies have been performed since the first commercial products came on the German market in the 1930s. Recent studies show that echinacea works best when taken at the very first sign of symptoms. Our experience shows that substantial and frequent doses are more likely to provide benefits. The strongest immune stimulation doesn't last more than 3 to 4 hours, so taking 2 droppersful of the tincture in water or tea every few hours will provide the strongest benefits. Clinical studies are variable: some show that echinacea preparations work well, and others show no effect. The dose, freshness of the herb, quality of the product, and frequency and quantity of dosing, along with your immune status, diet, and how much sleep you get, all play crucial roles in its effectiveness.

Echinacea preparations have also been widely recommended for treating skin conditions and infections of all kinds: spider bites; wasp, bee, and ant stings; animal bites; viral infections, including the prevention and shortening of herpes outbreaks; and skin infections like boils and carbuncles. Be sure to use echinacea to treat and prevent infections from wounds: You should apply it externally as a compress or in a salve or cream, and take the tincture or tea internally at the same time. Capsules and tablets are also available, but these are less effective, in our opinion. Use the tincture in sprays for sore throats. Mouthwashes, toothpastes, and soaps that contain echinacea may be worth a try, as well.

Sambucus nigra,
ssp. *canadensis/caerulea,*
syn. *S. nigra, S. canadensis,*
S. mexicana

Family: Adoxaceae

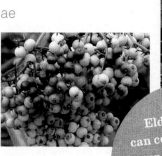

Elder

Elder flowers can cool and gently lower fevers, and the fruit is a classic medicine for flu symptoms.

Native and widespread, the compounds from the flowers and berries of the herbalist's beloved elder, a virtual medicine chest, are found in a range of commercial products. Elder has long held a hallowed status in Europe, where in some regions it is historically known as the home of the Elder Mother—the queenly figure who rules over the garden in the land of fairies—and it is also remembered as the source material for Pan's pipes. (The name *Sambucus* derives from the Greek word for a flute made of elder's hollow stems.)

Description

This large shrub or small tree has masses of fragrant, creamy yellow, umbrella-shaped flowers that mature into dark blue or black berries. If you're gathering from a similar plant that has red berries, you have *S. racemosa* (red elder); do not harvest from it, as its fruits are considered toxic and are best avoided.

Preparations and Dosage

For colds, flu, and fever, take 1 to 2 cups of the flower infusion two or three times daily (or as needed) to induce sweating, promote cleansing, and reduce heat. Pour 1 cup of boiling water over 2 tablespoons of fresh or dried elder blossoms, infuse for 10 minutes, and strain. You can also use 1 to 2 droppersful of the tincture in lemon balm, yarrow, peppermint, or any other pleasant tea of your choice.

Be sure to make elderberry syrup and elderberry jelly; they're both healing and delicious. You'll find elder syrups in natural food stores; follow the label instructions. Elder flower wines and cordials are also traditional.

Healing Properties

Historically and today, elder flowers and fruit are considered the premier herbs to use in preparations for the prevention and treatment of colds and, especially, flu. Some laboratory studies show elder fruit to have a powerful antiviral action. These purple berries are also loaded with anthocyanins, the same potent antioxidants found in grapes and blueberries.

Elder's antiviral properties make it effective at shortening and easing the symptoms of colds, flu, and fevers. Elder flowers make an excellent detoxifier and help treat inflammatory conditions and infections such as acne, boils, skin rashes, and dermatitis, especially when used periodically as part of a cleansing detoxification program. They have also long been recommended by herbalists to relieve hay fever and sinusitis, chronic rheumatism, neuralgia, and sciatica. The berries strengthen resistance to infections by supporting immune function.

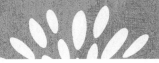

Safety

There are no safety concerns. However, do not confuse the medicinal elder with red elder (*S. racemosa*), and do not consume too many *raw* berries, to avoid diarrhea or digestive upset.

In the Garden

You'll get better flower and berry production if you grow elder in full sun, but it can also do well in partial shade in hot areas. It is fast growing and can shoot up more than 4 feet yearly if given rich soil, regular moisture, and plenty of drainage. If not, it's adaptable. A moderate pruning every 3 or 4 years during the dormant season helps to renew and strengthen elder's vigor. Propagate it by seed, stem cuttings, or root suckers. The seed is a multicycle germinator, so if you plant in late summer and let it overwinter, you'll have germination in the spring. Use composted, nonsterile soil. Cuttings are super easy to propagate: Take stem cuttings in spring or summer and hardwood cuttings in late fall.

Harvesting Elder: Be sure to gather the flowers after the morning dew has dried. If the flowers are compressed when wet, they'll blacken quickly, and they'll ferment if not promptly refrigerated. Handle them gently, as they bruise easily. You won't get an appreciable harvest until the second or third year. When gathering the berries, cut the whole umbel when the fruits are juicy and dark blue to black, and loosen the individual berries with a fork. Cook, dry, or process them right away. If you're drying them, wait until they've finished before you remove the stems. Be sure to give them air space: The flowers brown and bruise easily, and the berries can stick together and mold.

Foeniculum vulgare

Family: Apiaceae

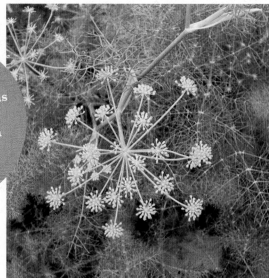

Fennel's golden, anise-flavored seeds help prevent gas and aid digestion after a meal.

Fennel

Don't be fooled by the name: This is not Florence fennel (*F. vulgare* var. *dulce*), which is grown for its edible bulb (botanically, that bulb is actually the swollen stem) and is found in the produce aisle. In this case, you're looking for the leaf or, more commonly, the seeds of a roadside wanderer that's used to flavor pickles, liqueurs, breads, and candies. Lest you think fennel a common weed, however, consider its pedigree: Legend has it that the knowledge of the Greek gods was delivered to mankind by Mercury, the messenger, as a burning coal in a fennel stalk.

Description

Native to the Mediterranean, fennel has made itself at home in dry, temperate areas here in the United States. It is a tall perennial, growing to 8 feet, with delicious, anise-flavored, lacy, divided leaves and bright yellow umbrella-shaped flowerheads, where the sweet seeds develop. It is a virtual maelstrom of pollinator activity when it's in flower, and green-and-yellow–striped swallowtail caterpillars consider it their diet of choice.

Preparations and Dosage

Make the tea by simmering 1 teaspoon of the seeds for each cup of water for 5 minutes. Remove it from the heat and let it stand, covered, for another 20 minutes before straining the seeds (if desired). Drink 1 cup before meals as needed. You can also take 3 or 4 capsules at a time, but then you will miss out on the wonderfully refreshing and sweet taste of the tea. Fennel seeds can be found in little dishes—along with shredded coconut and tiny "good and plenty" candies—on the front counters of many Indian restaurants, as they've traditionally been used in Middle Eastern cultures to prevent and relieve gas and indigestion after a hearty meal.

Healing Properties

Fennel seeds, known for their pleasant licorice or anise taste, make a great tea, addition to tincture formulas, and ingredient in soups, stews, and salads. You can also use the leaf as a culinary herb while you're waiting for the flowers to appear in late summer. (The leaves lose their juiciness as the plants bloom.)

The fresh or dried seeds have long been a popular remedy for dyspepsia, flatulence, nausea, stomachache, and the pains and spasms of colic and diarrhea in babies and young children. Fennel has been used for centuries to increase lactation. Fennel seed preparations, including teas, are used worldwide to stimulate digestion and appetite, help ease the symptoms of bronchitis and coughs, and flavor medicines. The essential oil eases muscular and rheumatic pains.

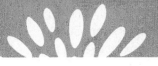

Safety

There are no concerns of note. Fennel has been used in cooking for many centuries.

People with a known sensitivity to anethole (the constituent responsible for fennel's milk-promoting activity in mothers) should avoid the seeds, though this condition is rare. Mild estrogenic activity has been noted in the essential oil and the tincture, so it's best to avoid these during pregnancy or nursing, but drinking the tea is perfectly safe.

In the Garden

Fennel seed will sprout in the garden readily, as long as the soil is warm. You can broadcast it directly at any time of year: It is quite a spreader and will pop up everywhere. Disturbed or poor soil is fine, and once fennel is established, no further watering or care is necessary. Plant in full sun to assure that the seeds mature quickly—otherwise, they may not ripen before winter weather causes them to mold. Just clear the dieback in the winter in preparation for next year's spring growth. If you get consistent winter snow, you'll grow fennel as an annual.

Harvesting Fennel: Gather the leaves at any time of year, but preferably before seed production begins, after which the leaves are tougher and sparser. Harvest seeds when they are turning from green to yellowish brown. Some say the seed is sweeter in younger plants. You can snip whole umbels and then rub the seeds off with your fingers. Some people riddle (rub) the ripening seedheads on hardware cloth propped over a basket or bowl. If you want to store dried seeds, harvest them when they are plump but still green, and air-dry them.

Allium sativum

Family: Amaryllidaceae, formerly Alliaceae

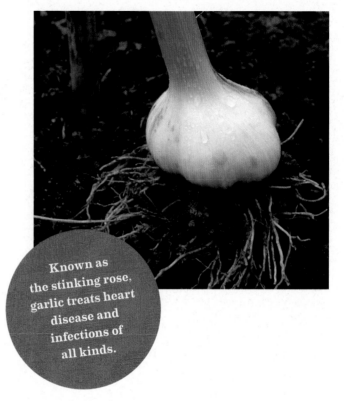

Known as the stinking rose, garlic treats heart disease and infections of all kinds.

Garlic

Who needs an introduction to this "stinking rose"? We just need to grow a steady supply of it, whether it's to repel vampires or cure a cold. Some people believe that garlic may be the oldest cultivated plant known to humankind; its use by Egyptian pyramid workers 3 millennia ago was mentioned in ancient writings. Don't worry about garlic affecting your breath, though; just remember to relay all the benefits of garlic to your friends, and you'll soon be in good company!

Description

The bulb is well known—it's creamy white, has a papery membrane, and is composed of a number of similarly papered "cloves." Above ground, it has round, hollow leaves and purple, umbrella-shaped flowering parts. The leaves usually die down in midsummer to late summer.

Preparations and Dosage

When you've eaten all of the garlic you've grown in your garden, head to the supermarket. It's available in the produce aisle, and also in capsules and tablets (some of which are odor-free), powders, and oils. Eat 2 to 3 cloves daily with meals, or take 2 to 4 perles of a garlic product daily. Better yet, take your homemade garlic syrup!

Healing Properties

Garlic is warming, or activating, to the digestive and respiratory tracts, and it has pronounced antibiotic and antiviral effects. It has a long history of use to help prevent parasites of the colon and promote good digestion. Herbalists like to use the crushed bulb, primarily raw, in syrups and stirred into soups for fighting colds, flu, bronchitis, pneumonia, and other infections. Mixing it with foods prevents the raw garlic from causing digestive upset and nausea, and adding it at the end of the cooking process will preserve its medicinal potency. When you're cooking or baking with garlic, make sure to crush the cloves first. Once the cells are crushed, an enzyme is released that produces the main active compound, allicin, which then breaks down into other active compounds. If the cloves are cooked before crushing, much of this important enzyme is lost.

Another reason to eat garlic regularly is to promote good cardiovascular health. Some studies show that garlic can help balance cholesterol and provide other health benefits, including cancer prevention. Garlic has a mild platelet-stabilizing effect, which may help prevent abnormal clotting and reduce the risk of stroke and heart attack, especially when used regularly.

Safety

Avoid garlic if you're nursing, as the taste can be transmitted to breast milk. Raw cloves can sometimes irritate your stomach and cause nausea if eaten on an empty stomach, but cooking reduces much of garlic's irritating and warming qualities.

Some researchers advise caution when ingesting garlic immediately before or after surgery and with anticoagulant drugs.

In the Garden

Place individual cloves 1 to 2 inches deep in rich soil with the pointed tips up, in September or October, and let them overwinter under mulch. During the growing season, full sun is best and nitrogen fertilizer is helpful. For the strongest garlic flavor, medicinal strength, and biggest bulbs, remove the flowering stalks as they form. Keep the soil moist until you notice that the tops are beginning to yellow, and then stop watering.

Harvesting Garlic: The best time to harvest the bulbs is in summer, after the tops have died down. When the leaves turn yellow and fall over, the bulbs are ready. Dig them, resist the urge to wash them (just brush off any excess dirt), and tie a small group together by their stems. Hang the groups in a dark, dry location with good air circulation, or lay them on screens or lattice to dry. As they dry, the skins will become papery and the color will mellow. They'll be at their best after a week or two. Store garlic in a dark spot, in a breathable container.

Centella asiatica,
syn. *Hydrocotyle asiatica*

Family: Apiaceae

This tropical weedy herb is an ingredient in popular health drinks that aid in mental clarity.

Gotu kola

Introduced from the Indian subtropics, gotu kola is used as food for meditation by yogis and is one of the most important herbs in that country's Ayurvedic medical tradition. According to legend, elephants are blessed with good memories as a result of their consumption of gotu kola in the jungle. You'll see pushcart vendors juicing the leaves and selling the beverage throughout many parts of southeast Asia, attesting to its reputation as a "supreme" herb that awakens the crown chakra and confers long life.

Description

A creeping and spreading herbaceous tender perennial with round, tender leaves and trailing stems, gotu kola has a pleasant, sweet-and-sour taste and a crunchy texture. The green to lavender flowers are barely noticeable under the leaves. Gotu kola is frost tender, so it is grown indoors or as an annual in all but the warmest, most humid climates.

Preparations and Dosage

Positive clinical studies have typically used a dose of 60 to 120 milligrams, and up to 500 milligrams (for its anti-anxiety effects), twice daily, of the standardized extract in capsule or tablet form. Commercial products typically contain 100 to 300 milligrams per capsule or tablet.

Clinical studies have been conducted using the herb extract, but regular use of the plant's juice or leaves in salads and cooking can provide similar, though milder, benefits. Juice gotu kola with other vegetables, such as celery (great taste!), add the leaves to salads and other dishes for daily use, or make teas or tinctures from the leaves or whole plant.

Healing Properties

Besides the traditional reputation of gotu kola for improving and preserving memory, mental function, and longevity, clinical studies indicate that it can provide real benefits for cardiovascular health, diabetes, and oral and gum health, as well as reduce anxiety and nervousness.

Studies have shown that gotu kola extract can benefit the circulation in diabetics and shorten the time it takes to heal diabetic ulcers. This same attribute helps diabetics and nondiabetics alike to reduce their risk of hypertension and abnormal clotting and plaque formation in the blood vessels. Other studies have supported the traditional uses of gotu kola and shown that the extract helps reduce anxiety and improve memory and mood.

Gotu kola preparations are thought to clear toxins and reduce inflammation, helping to ease the symptoms of rheumatism and rheumatoid arthritis. The juice or leaves can also be used to stimulate your appetite when needed and promote good digestion.

You can make or buy creams containing the extract to heal eczema, wounds, and other skin conditions. The herb has been shown to stimulate the production of collagen and to help improve the tone of veins near the surface of your skin.

Safety

Gotu kola has been used as a common culinary green in Asia for centuries, and it is considered to have low toxicity.

In the Garden

This beautiful creeper prefers warm, moist, humid conditions. In most zones, it will never see the outside of your sun-porch or greenhouse. If you want to grow it outside for part of the year, it's a good choice for a pot or planter. In four-season climates, you can bring it indoors for the winter if you can provide a deep container in a humid greenhouse or atrium. Gotu kola needs rich soil and lots of nutrition, especially nitrogen-rich fertilizer. Mist it daily so it gets adequate humidity. If you can grow it outside, place it in full sun or partial shade, depending on the aridity it will encounter, and leave lots of space for it to expand, as it spreads by runners. It is not easy to start from seed—in the best warm and moist conditions, it will still take more than a month to germinate—so if you can get a cutting or a root division, you're in luck.

Harvesting Gotu Kola: You can use the leaves or the whole plant, discarding any yellowing leaves as you harvest. If you can give the plant a moist, warm environment and collect only leaves, you'll get lots of grow-back, possibly year-round. If you harvest the whole plant, just be sure to clean it well. Dry it as quickly as possible, but not with high heat, as it has a tendency to turn brown.

Crataegus laevigata,
C. oxycantha,
and C. pinnatifida

Family: Rosaceae

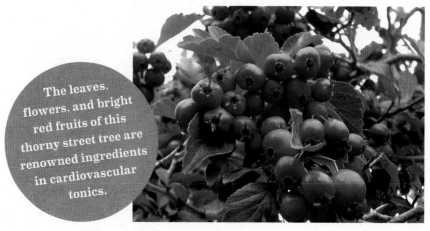

The leaves, flowers, and bright red fruits of this thorny street tree are renowned ingredients in cardiovascular tonics.

Hawthorn

For strength, beauty, and a sense of tradition, along with a wonderful complement of healing powers, the hawthorn tree stands by itself. It has appeared in Greek and European poetry, art, and literature from earliest times, a symbol of hope and love. The branches were cut down at night on the eve of May to be incorporated into the maypole and May Day rituals, and for that reason it was called the "mayflower." But perhaps its most lasting legacy lives on in the name of the ship the Pilgrims sailed across the Atlantic for the New World, endowing it with their finest wishes and dreams for the future.

Description

Hawthorn is a small- to medium-size thorny tree or large shrub with dark, glossy, green, toothed or lobed leaves. Clusters of white, pink, or crimson flowers appear in the spring, and deep red berries follow in the fall. Two hundred species occur worldwide, and most can be used medicinally, although a large number are ornamental hybrids. The species we've listed above are well established for medicine making.

Preparations and Dosage

The recommended dosage is 2 to 3 droppersful of the tincture in water, 1 cup of the tea (made from the leaf and flower and/or fruit), or 3 or 4 capsules of the powdered extract, two or three times daily. Or, take 1 tablespoon of the syrup twice daily and spread your toast with hawthorn berry jam. (You can make your own from the red, ripe fruits.) You'll find hawthorn in natural food stores as liquid tinctures, tablets, capsules, and syrups, and also in traditional Chinese herb shops in wafer form (called "haw flakes").

Healing Properties

The leaf and flower have traditionally been used in Europe to promote heart health. European doctors and herbalists alike frequently recommend hawthorn preparations for anyone with cardiovascular problems, especially in the beginning stages of disease. This includes hypertension, cholesterol imbalances, heartbeat irregularities, and even congestive heart failure, where hawthorn acts to strengthen the heart's pumping action. Flavonoids and other powerful antioxidants in hawthorn can help protect your heart and promote cardiovascular health. It can be used regularly, even for years. Hawthorn is also commonly known to reduce anxiety and nervousness, benefitting insomnia and calming a racing mind. For thousands of years, the large, glossy, red fruits of the Chinese hawthorn (*C. pinnatifida*) have been an important remedy in traditional Chinese medicine for preventing and treating bloating, stomach distention, and difficulty in digesting fatty foods.

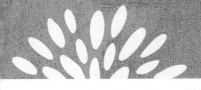

Safety

Most worries about hawthorn's safety are theoretical, but it can potentiate (strengthen) the effects of digitalis medications, although these are not commonly prescribed in modern medical practice. If you are taking beta-blockers or other drugs for high blood pressure, or if you have very low blood pressure, talk with your doctor or experienced natural-care practitioner or herbalist before taking hawthorn.

In the Garden

In their native temperate zones, these shrubby trees occur near stream flats, meadows, woods, and forests, so they prefer a location that is sunny to partially shaded, with nutrient-rich, loamy, alkaline soil. If you buy a small tree, water it deeply when establishing it. You can propagate hawthorn by seed, but be aware that it has complex dormancy needs. The seed must be washed and stratified or soaked in water for 2 to 3 days, then the pulp must be removed and the seed sown immediately. Hawthorn is a slow germinator and takes a minimum of 6 months, and up to 18 months, to emerge. Propagation by cuttings from a friend's tree (or, easier yet, root suckers) can be a much easier way to go!

Harvesting Hawthorn: Harvest the leaves and flowers early in the flowering stage with minimal stem attached; harvest the mature red berries in the fall after the first frost, but before repeated frost or freezing destroys their firmness. Give the fruits and flowers plenty of room for air circulation when drying, and dry the berry whole, as this enables it to remain stable for several years.

Lonicera japonica

Family: Adoxaceae,
syn. Caprifoliaceae

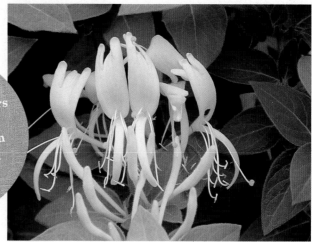

The fragrant, nectar-filled flowers and stems of honeysuckle form a living fence in the garden.

Honeysuckle

This lovely, cascading, woody vine, with its divine scent, is often planted as a landscape attraction. It dazzles the eye with its gorgeous blooms in warm weather and retreats to a pleasant but unremarkable placeholder at other times of the year. Its name refers to the fact that fairies (and everyone else) love to sip the nectar from the flowers. There are well over 100 different species, and at least 15 are used medicinally.

Description

Honeysuckle is a perennial, deciduous or evergreen climbing shrub that typically wraps tightly around other plants or a support. It can grow to over 20 feet long and is invasive enough to be considered a noxious weed in the eastern United States. The tubular flowers bloom in the summer and are a pale yellow, sometimes tinged with pink, that turns a darker golden color as they age. Orangish red fruits that are rather nasty-tasting but are attractive to birds occur in clusters following the flowers in the fall.

Preparations and Dosage

Make a strong infusion by steeping the flowers for as long as 30 minutes, or even gently simmering them, and drink $1/2$ to 1 cup twice daily, or as often as desired. Honeysuckle also makes a delicious syrup. It's found commercially in powder, granule, extract, and tablet form. Follow the directions on the product label.

Healing Properties

The flowers (or the flowers plus young stems) are mildly antibiotic and antiviral and are used to treat colds and flu. They are also recommended in traditional Chinese medicine (TCM) for relief of upper respiratory tract infections, fevers, bronchitis, sore throat, heat stroke, and diarrhea. The tea is also known for healing boils and other skin infections, as it helps to remove "fire toxins" (a TCM description that refers to metabolic waste buildup and inflammation) from your body. Teenagers and anyone who is prone to acne, boils, and sties can drink the refreshing tea daily to reap the strongest benefits.

Western herbalists recommend taking the flower tea or extract to relieve hot flashes, to prevent and promote healing of urinary tract infections, and to treat skin conditions like acne, boils, and eczema. The whole vine, including the leaves and twigs, can be decocted and used as a compress for treating burns, sores, and acne.

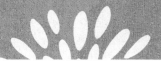

Safety

The flowers and twigs are considered nontoxic by traditional Chinese medical practitioners.

In the Garden

Honeysuckle is frost hardy, heat tolerant, and sturdy; it's an easy plant to have around. If you want to create a hedge or fencerow, plant honeysuckle vines 3 feet apart, and expect them to push those bounds unless you trim them back during the dormant season. Honeysuckle likes moist, rich soil but is adaptable and somewhat drought tolerant once it's large, and it will do well in full sun (or even partial shade, in hot climates). Start it from seed, if you're willing to wait a month or two for germination (stratification helps), or take stem cuttings in the spring or woody cuttings in the fall. Easier yet, try layering a neighbor's plant. Be sure to provide a trellis or fence for it to climb. Stems will trail along the ground, and you may want to prune them back for a tidier look.

Harvesting Honeysuckle:

Collect the flowers when they are just starting to open and are lovely, fresh, and have a creamy hue. (Older, orange flowers will dry to a brown color.) Be sure to pick them every few days. As with all flowers, honeysuckle blooms are fragile and will bruise easily, so gather them in the morning, before the warmth of the day has compromised their freshness. Dry them immediately after harvest, at a low temperature and out of the sun. Tender stems may be collected also; they contain many of the same compounds.

Humulus lupulus

Family: Cannabidaceae

The flowers of this plant give beer and ale their bitter flavors and are widely used as an anti-inflammatory.

Hops

Known worldwide as the main flavoring agent in beers and ales, the flowering cones of this scabrous (rough-textured) plant were once prescribed by British physicians to King George III for his insomnia and stuffed into a pillow to promote sleep for their royal patient. These days, you'll find many varieties selected specifically for brewing purposes.

Description

This deer-resistant perennial vine will grow to 30 feet long, leaping over and engulfing other plants, and can be found on tall supports throughout hops-growing regions around the world. Its green leaves and stems are rough and sandpapery, with razor-sharp hairs. The strobiles (the female conelike flowering parts) develop in late summer, turning from green to yellow and finally drying to brown. These same strobiles produce a very bitter golden yellow resinous powder called lupulin, which is considered the most important medicinal substance in the plant.

Preparations and Dosage

Hops makes a good tincture because the resinous yellow lupulin in the female flowers is more soluble in alcohol than it is in water. Use ¼ to ½ teaspoon at a time in a little water or tea, two or three times a day.

Hops extracts, including standardized extracts, are available in capsules and tablets. Follow the label directions.

You can sew dried hops strobiles into small sacks and place them under your pillow to promote sound sleep, or you can add hops tea to your bathwater.

Healing Properties

Hops is famous for promoting sleep and relaxation and for imparting a refreshing bitter taste to beer and ale. Specifically, herbalists recommend hops for allaying nervousness, restlessness, excitability, heart palpitations, nervous digestion, and insomnia. Midwives have used preparations of hops for increasing the flow of new mothers' milk.

Recent research has shown that hops extracts have strong anti-inflammatory and pain-relieving actions for arthritis and other inflammatory conditions. Hops also has estrogenic action, which has been cited as the reason why men who drink excessive amounts of very hoppy beer or ale can develop noticeable breasts.

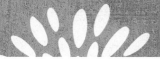

Safety

Some herbalists feel that it is wise to avoid using hops if you are depressed, for fear that the sedative could accentuate this mood state. Also, a purely theoretical interaction has been suggested between hops and pharmaceutical sedatives or painkillers.

Handle hops carefully, as the pollen can cause a skin rash. We don't consider moderate hops use during pregnancy to be a problem, though some have contraindicated it because of its known (though mild) estrogenic effects.

In the Garden

Hops needs full sun; deep, rich soil; mulch; and warmth; and it benefits from nitrogen-rich fertilizer. If you're transplanting it into your garden, make sure the soil has warmed up first. It is drought tolerant once established. Give it a fence or trellis, and space your plants 3 to 6 feet apart. It can also be container grown and can climb up any support you provide. Starting it from seed is difficult because germination is usually quite low, though stratifying helps, as does overnight soaking. The best ways to propagate are to take cuttings (including at least two sets of buds on each one), pulling up stems that have layered, or dividing the root, which is the easiest and usually most successful option. In mild climates, the plant spreads easily by root runners after a few years.

Harvesting Hops: Pick the strobiles in autumn on a clear, dry day when they begin to feel slightly papery and firm and are turning amber in color. They will deteriorate if not dried quickly. Store them carefully to prevent moisture from browning them after drying. Their potency fades quickly and shelf life is typically less than a year. You can also freeze fresh hops, if you wish.

Lavandula angustifolia

Family: Lamiaceae

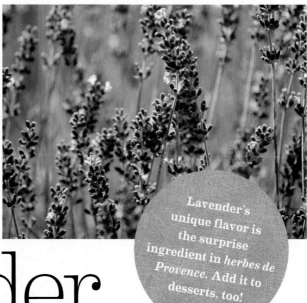

Lavender's unique flavor is the surprise ingredient in herbes de Provence. Add it to desserts, too!

Lavender

The stuff of legends, lavender figures in story, song, and fantasy. It is so very versatile: a culinary, cosmetic, and medicinal herb all in one, and a universally loved fragrance, as well! But be sure you are purchasing and growing the lavender you really want. There is a dizzying array of lavenders for you to choose from, including lavandin, sometimes erroneously called French lavender (*L. x intermedia*), Spanish lavender (*L. stoechas*), and French lavender (*L. dentata*). All of them, though notable in their own rights, are but a distraction from the beloved medicinal English lavender.

Description

This deer-resistant midsize shrub, with its aromatic grey-green upright foliage and tall purple flowers on tapering, pointed spikes, is familiar to us all. It is perennial in warm to temperate climates and evergreen in warmer, drier ones. Lavandin, which is often substituted for and is hard to distinguish from English lavender, is taller, with a stronger, spicier aroma.

Preparations and Dosage

Make an infusion and drink 1 cup two or three times daily. Use 1 dropperful of the tincture in tea or water to take advantage of the relaxing and uplifting effects.

Add a few drops of lavender essential oil to a bottle of unscented massage oil (let your nose be your guide when deciding how much to add) for an enhanced body treatment. Incorporate this scented oil into steams, wraps, compresses, inhalers, and baths. It is divine in potpourris, and it can be used to flavor desserts and confections, as well.

Healing Properties

The flowering spikes, leaves, and young stems are harvested and dried, and then the volatiles (the aromatic chemicals) are extracted to produce lavender oil. Lavender oil is a staple for aromatherapy and internal use, and the flavor and fragrance industries make use of it in cosmetics, shampoos, bath salts, and a myriad of other products.

Aside from the oil, lavender flowers are found in teas, tinctures, and extracts, and they're recommended by herbalists to lift the spirits; relax the body; allay nausea, digestive upset, and colic; and promote a relaxing sleep.

Lavender broadly strengthens the nervous system and is recommended for stress headaches and nervous exhaustion. It can also help relieve flatulence, intestinal spasms, and colic. Laboratory studies have shown that lavender has anti-inflammatory and sedative effects. These come primarily from one of its major constituents, linalool, which is a well-known calmative.

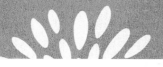

Safety

There are no real concerns. The oil can occasionally cause allergic reactions with repeated use, and the internal use of lavender can cause a mild allergenic effect in sensitive people, but both occurrences are very rare. There are no contraindications for using lavender teas or tinctures during pregnancy and lactation, but the oil should be used with caution during those times, as should most essential oils.

In the Garden

Lavenders are native to the Mediterranean and Middle Eastern regions, except for lavandin, which is a recent hybrid. English lavender (*L. angustifolia*) should be your choice for medicinal and cosmetic use, and like the other lavenders, it loves full sun and well-drained, gravelly soil. Its roots rot in wet soil and it doesn't do well in areas with high humidity. The more compact 'Munstead' and 'Hidcote' varieties overwinter best. In desert regions, however, lavender may need some summer water in very sandy soil. In warm climates, you will want to prune it back after flowering and once again to a mounded shape during the dormant season (late winter or early spring). Prune only to greenery, not into the woody stems. In four-season areas, clip it back moderately after flowering, and give it a severe shaping, down to the lowest greenery but not into the woody stems, as temperatures begin to warm in the spring. Protect the plant from winter winds and freezing temperatures. Cuttings are best for propagation (taking care that your medium doesn't become waterlogged), since the seed does not germinate easily and lavender doesn't always produce true to form. You can also trying propagating by layering.

Harvesting Lavender: Gather the buds just as the flowers are beginning to open on a dry, warm, sunny morning. (Cold or rainy weather will lower the essential oil content.) Separate the flowers from the stems after they are dry—not before—to avoid bruising them.

Melissa officinalis

Family: Lamiaceae

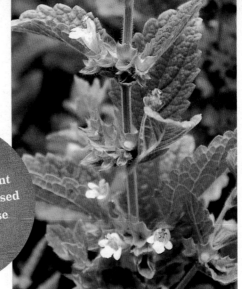

The "gladdening herb" is an ancient monastery herb used to calm and ease fevers and agitation.

Lemon balm

Once used to polish furniture and named *Melissa* (which means "honeybee" in Latin) because of its ability to attract bees and reportedly keep them from absconding from the hive, lemon balm's oils are refreshing both externally and internally. It has the distinction of being one of the safest garden herbs to use for health, and it's also one of the best tasting. This European favorite was grown in monastery gardens and made into elixirs and magical brews in the Middle Ages, through the Renaissance, and to the present. It is sometimes called the "gladdening herb" because it lifts the spirits.

Description

This delightfully scented herbaceous perennial has lush green, textured, aromatic foliage and a delicate habit. It enjoys a wide range of conditions, grows to 2 feet tall with wide-spreading branches, and self-seeds profusely in the garden.

Preparations and Dosage

Lemon balm works best in teas and tonic elixirs, where its uplifting scent and taste can titillate your senses with its relaxing lemon fragrance. Put a few sprigs of lemon balm in a pitcher of water and leave it in the fridge to infuse over a couple of days. Enjoy this as a cool summer drink.

Make an infusion and drink 2 or 3 cups daily or when needed. You can also make creams, salves, and ointments for skin complaints.

Healing Properties

Lemon balm is refreshing and relaxing, settling both the stomach and the nerves. Herbalists recommend it for calming a nervous heart and counteracting tension and insomnia, as well as for relaxing spasms of the stomach and intestines. As a tea sipped after meals, it can also ease heartburn and relieve digestive upsets, such as a feeling of pressure or distension in the abdomen.

Lemon balm has antiviral properties, and in the case of such viral conditions as herpes outbreaks, you can drink the tea throughout the day and before bedtime. The phenolic fraction (a group of chemicals that have strong antioxidant properties), which can be extracted from the plant by gently simmering the whole herb for 40 to 60 minutes, is effective at relieving the pain and duration of herpes sores.

The cooled tea infusion of the herb can be given to infants and young children by the spoonful to relieve colic and restlessness. It is the only herb we found that we had both needed when our infant children experienced difficult colic, crying, and restlessness during their first years.

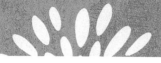

Safety

No concerns are known.

In the Garden

Lemon balm is very adaptable: It does well in full sun, but in the hottest areas, partial shade may be preferable. It is frost hardy and tolerates crowding, as well as rich or poor soil. It prefers moist soil with good drainage, but it will develop higher amounts of the medicinal constituents when subjected to some water stress. Waterlogged soil will often cause the plant to die back. Lemon balm will self-sow and spread easily, but if you want to start it from seed, do so in early spring in cool soil, whether indoors or out. (Stratification is beneficial.) You can also easily start it from cuttings or divide and replant the roots.

Harvesting Lemon Balm: Gather healthy leaves (discard any that are yellowing) and flexible stems from early to full bloom in midsummer, and again in late summer to early fall. The essential oil content is highest in late bloom. Do not harvest when the leaves are wet, and be careful not to bruise them. They dry easily and quickly, but need total darkness. Also, don't pile them thickly, and remember that if they are bruised or heated up during harvesting, they will blacken during drying. Lemon balm has a short shelf life in storage.

Aloysia citriodora,
syn. A. triphylla

Family: Verbenaceae

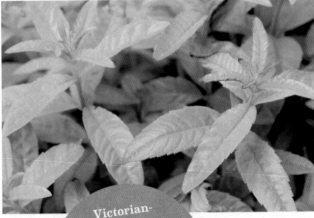

Victorian-era Europeans believed in the power of this herb's perfume to induce passion in anyone who sniffed it.

Lemon verbena

A sweeter scent in the garden you'll never know! No wonder it was used in perfumeries in medieval times. Lemon verbena was brought to Spain from Chile and Peru in the late 1700s, and *Aloysia* refers to Spain's much-beloved queen, Maria Luisa, wife of King Charles IV, who favored this herb. Besides its delightful aroma and flavor, the tea has decidedly beneficial qualities as a strong antioxidant and relaxing herb.

Description

In very warm climates, this aromatic deer-resistant plant can achieve a height of 10 feet and remain evergreen year-round, but in most areas it will die back each winter, and in four-season zones it's usually grown as an annual. Lemon verbena is shrubby, with rough, lance-shaped leaves that are arranged in whorled threes and are almost oily to the touch. Whitish pink flowers burst from the tops of the stems.

Preparations and Dosage

Make an infusion and drink 1 cup several times a day and before bedtime. You can add honey to the tea and mix it into fruit salads for a sparkling taste treat and added health benefits. Use lemon verbena in potpourris, and soak the dried or fresh herb in the liquid portion of a cake or custard batter before completing the recipe.

Dried lemon verbena leaves can also be included in a sachet and added to a hot bath for a relaxing and refreshing soak.

Healing Properties

Many studies have shown that lemon verbena contains strong antioxidants. When the extract was given to male runners, it helped to speed muscle recovery and protect their tissues against oxidative damage during repeated running sessions. Traditionally, lemon verbena tea or extract has been used to aid digestion, promote sleep, and act as a mild sedative or calmative.

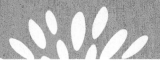

Safety

Regular long-term use may cause indigestion or upset stomach in some people, but this is rare. When used externally, the essential oil may cause photosensitivity in some individuals.

In the Garden

Lemon verbena enjoys full sun and rich soil. Mulch it to conserve moisture, water it well, and let the soil dry out between waterings. (It is sensitive to fungus, so do not overwater.) This plant is deciduous in all but the hottest areas, but you can take it inside for the winter and keep it evergreen if you give it supplemental lighting. If you live in a four-season climate, you can also try placing it in a big pot against a warm southern wall during the summer months and wintering it indoors. It's easy to propagate from cuttings, but the seed needs warm temperatures, and germination rates are typically low.

Harvesting Lemon Verbena: Gather the leaves and the stem (if it's the top flexible portion), with or without flowers. Be very gentle when handling the leaves, as they bruise easily and consequently brown or blacken during drying. To dry, you might want to harvest long stems and use the hang method and separate the leaves after they've dried. Watch that they don't overdry: It's easy to do, and if it happens the essential oils will be lost. Store lemon verbena leaves in a dark place or an opaque container, since they are sensitive to light.

Glycyrrhiza glabra,
G. uralensis

Family: Fabaceae

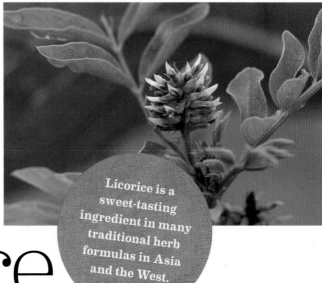

Licorice is a sweet-tasting ingredient in many traditional herb formulas in Asia and the West.

Licorice

Licorice sticks, licorice whips, licorice jelly beans . . . nowadays these treats are probably flavored with less-expensive anise oil. Even so, the sweet root of this plant is still used in commerce. Licorice has figured prominently in traditional Chinese medicine for 5,000 years, and it was even found in the tomb of King Tutankhamen of Egypt. One of its constituents, a substance called glycyrrhizin, is 50 times sweeter than table sugar. That's why it's used so extensively in traditional Chinese medicine—it "harmonizes" the other herbs. This may simply be a euphemism for "makes the medicine go down," and you might agree, after tasting some other Chinese herbs!

Description

This spiky perennial is in the pea family and has the characteristic look: pinnately compound leaves on a long stalk with lavender to purple pea-like flowers. The creeping rhizomes sometimes reach 12 feet or more in length, and after several years may pop up far away from the original plant.

Preparations and Dosage

Licorice is found in many kinds of preparations—teas, syrups, tinctures, elixirs, lozenges, drinks, and food products.

To make a decoction at home, simmer the roots for 30 to 45 minutes longer than usual and then strain them out. Drink ½ cup of the liquid two or three times daily for the conditions indicated.

Licorice is most often blended with other herbs, though it can be used by itself for digestive and respiratory tract symptoms.

Natural food stores carry numerous licorice products in powder, granule, capsule, and tablet forms. Follow the directions on the product label.

Healing Properties

Licorice is an amazingly versatile herb. Besides imparting a sweet taste to often unpleasant-tasting herbal formulas, it is used to treat inflammation and irritation of the respiratory, urinary, and digestive tracts. Licorice has decidedly soothing, anti-inflammatory, and antiviral effects. As a tea, tincture, syrup, or standardized extract, it has often been recommended for soothing and helping to heal stomach ulcers and inflammatory bowel and liver conditions. The root is also an excellent expectorant, which is why it's often recommended for easing the symptoms of respiratory tract infections, including coughs, sore throats, and excess phlegm and congestion. Licorice preparations are also recommended by herbalists for helping to counteract stress and fatigue, reportedly by supporting adrenal function.

Safety

Licorice causes your body to increase potassium excretion while simultaneously retaining sodium, which can affect blood pressure in some sensitive individuals. If you have moderate to major hypertension, it's best to avoid this herb. You can also supplement with extra potassium or eat potassium-rich greens daily during extended therapeutic use. The standard English language *Materia Medica* for Chinese herbs notes that licorice should not be used by those with edema, hypertension, hypokalemia (potassium deficiency), or congestive heart failure. Allergic reactions are infrequent but possible and usually take the form of a skin rash and digestive upset.

Some herbalists caution against the use of licorice during pregnancy, but many traditional Chinese herb sources do not.

In the Garden

In its native regions of the Mediterranean and southern China, licorice grows on grassy plains and scrublands in sunny, cool, dry spots. Licorice loves a sunny, cool, dry location in the garden, and it won't tolerate a soggy site or an extended hard freeze. The long taproots expand best in very loose, deep soil, but we've seen it become invasive in clay soils. Don't baby it with fertilizer if you want the best quality medicine; it will do best without added nutrients other than some lime or calcium, which it loves. If you want to keep it from flopping, provide a trellis or support. And expect it to spread by runners in a few years if it likes your care! The seed needs warm temperatures to germinate and appreciates either a soak in hot water or scarification. You can also divide the root into sections, making sure each section has one or two buds, and then plant them vertically. You can even replant the crown after you've harvested the root.

Harvesting Licorice: Gathering this herb requires a little planning because you'll dig the root in the fall or spring of its third or fourth year, and it's best if you don't let it flower the season before you harvest it. (Pinch back the buds if they appear.) The roots are usually cut vertically for drying. When you store licorice, keep in mind that it mildews easily and can attract insects.

Ligustrum lucidum

Family: Oleaceae

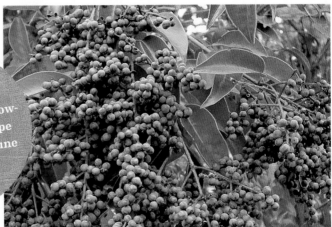

The ancients used the purple berries from this now-common landscape shrub as an immune and hormone tonic.

Ligustrum

This plant is also called Chinese privet or wax privet, and it's known in China as *Nu Zhen Zi*. Ligustrum is a very common landscape subject that is considered a weed in hot climates. You may even have removed one of its relatives when you were modernizing your garden! The dark purple fruits are attractive, and birds, especially cedar waxwings, flock to them. However, as common as ligustrum is, not many people know that the berries are a classic and widely used tonic herb in traditional Chinese medicine.

Description

Ligustrum is a shrub or tree with thick, glossy, dark green leaves and white flower clusters that give way to small, dark purple or blackish berries. It is sometimes pruned into hedges, which prevents it from forming berries, but if it is allowed to take on tree form, it can grow to 40 feet tall and, in warm climates, positively drip with fruit during the fall to winter months. However, don't confuse Chinese or Japanese privet with European privet (*L. vulgare*), which is mostly grown in hedge form and is reputed to be mildly toxic.

Preparations and Dosage

Make a tea by decocting the fresh or dried fruits for 40 to 60 minutes, and drink a cup two or three times each day. You can also make a dried tea concentrate and add ½ teaspoon of it to a little hot water to make an instant tea. Tinctures and syrups can be purchased, and many products in capsule and tablet form contain the herb. Follow the package instructions.

Healing Properties

Ligustrum berries are considered a premier tonic in Chinese herbal medicine. They are added to many formulas that treat chronic adrenal weakness due to stress and overwork, which is accompanied by symptoms such as low back pain, ringing in your ears, premature graying, blurry vision, and weakness in your legs.

Some studies show that the berries strengthen your immune system during cancer treatment and also act as an adaptogen, helping to beneficially regulate your hormonal and nervous system functions. Ligustrum is often recommended for long-term use in traditional Chinese herbal literature, especially for the elderly and for those who are run-down. The berries are also used to treat hot flashes, irritability, dizziness, and other liver-related deficiency symptoms.

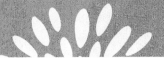

Safety

No concerns have been noted.

In the Garden

Ligustrum is typically hardy only in warm climates, but it will survive frosts and even occasional freezes. Within its range, your biggest concern will be how to manage it—sometimes you'll swear it grew 3 feet in a day. Don't trim it into a hedge, as this will eliminate the possibility that the plant will bear fruit. Instead, give it a lot of room to become a tree and commit to yearly pruning to keep the berries within reach. In four-season climates, you'll probably want to grow ligustrum in a pot and keep it sheltered from harsh weather. It is easy to grow from seed or stem cuttings, and it is readily available as a nursery plant. Full sun or partial shade is okay. The plant has no special soil requirements, and it's drought tolerant. Just remember that the dropped fruit can be messy and that the tree won't produce any until it is 4 or 5 years old.

Harvesting Ligustrum: Collect the berries when they have ripened to a dark bluish purple color, and wash and separate them promptly. Dry them thoroughly and slowly, so that they don't mold in storage.

Nigella damascena

Family: Ranunculaceae

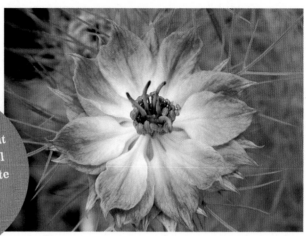

The seeds of this beautiful but short-lived annual are a culinary taste treat of orange and spice.

Love-in-a-mist

Love-in-a-mist and its closely related cousin black cumin (*N. sativa*) are ephemeral garden visitors, and these two species have been receiving attention because of the medicinal action of their seeds. Black cumin seeds, native to the Middle East and used there as a spice since ancient times, were found in the tomb of ancient Egypt's King Tutankhamen. The taste of the seeds of both species is enchanting—like a cross between mint, anise, and orange.

Description

These 6- to 12-inch annuals have sky blue to white five-petaled flowers, threadlike leaves, and ballooning seed capsules that dry and remain, skeletonlike, in the garden long after the green phase. Both plants tend to come and go before the heat of summer. They differ in the layering of the bracts on their flowering parts. Both have a distinctive "mist" of airy, petallike bracts and foliage, and both are found in a wide range of climates.

Preparations and Dosage

Combine 1 level teaspoon of the seed for each cup of freshly boiled water, and then let it steep for 15 to 20 minutes. Drink 1 cup of the tea several times a day. You can also make a tincture using a menstruum of 50 percent pure alcohol to 50 percent water, taking 1 to 2 droppersful in water or tea several times a day, or as needed.

As a spice, sprinkle the seeds liberally on bread dough before baking; into smoothies, soups, curries, and stews; and onto salads. The flowers are beautiful when added to floral arrangements, and the dried seedpods, if you have extras, make nice additions to dried arrangements.

Healing Properties

These two species of *Nigella* have a similar look and taste, but of the two, black cumin is the most studied, and according to some chemical analyses, it is also the stronger anti-inflammatory. It's likely that love-in-a-mist has similar properties, though they may be weaker.

The seeds of both contain healthful fatty acids such as linoleic acid, an aromatic volatile oil, and small amounts of other active substances.

Today, the seed of black cumin is a popular spice and medicine in parts of Asia and North Africa. It has a long history of traditional use that is well-documented in ancient texts. The seeds were eaten or decocted to ease stomach and gas pains; heal ulcers; and promote good respiratory tract, liver, kidney, and circulatory health. They were also taken when a diuretic was needed. Egyptians 3,000 years ago believed the seeds were a panacea, useful for any ailment. They were mentioned for healing in the Bible, and Mohammed was said to ingest them daily in honey. He reportedly said, "Use this seed often, as it is a cure for everything except death."

Recently, black cumin seed has undergone a worldwide resurgence in popularity. Both species have been noted to be antimicrobial, fever-lowering, pain-relieving, antioxidant, immune-activating, mildly estrogenic, anti-cancer, and cholesterol-lowering.

Safety

A review of a number of safety studies shows the whole seeds and extracts to be safe. Rarely, some people might experience a rash from handling the seeds. Eating a large amount of the raw seeds may upset your stomach, so lightly toast them before snacking on them, or add them to recipes to reduce that possibility.

In the Garden

These delicate annuals seem to come from another world! They are not really so much cultivated as hosted by gardeners, who are always eager for their springtime blessing. Both plants enjoy full sun and plenty of moisture, but not a waterlogged site. Easy to start from seed, love-in-a-mist and black cumin will happily return year after year unless they're weeded out successfully before they drop their seeds. Direct-seed them only, either in fall or very early spring, and if you want continual bloom, reseed every 3 to 4 weeks until summer's heat discourages their germination.

Harvesting Love-in-a-Mist and Black Cumin: When the seed capsules have matured and browned, break them open and collect the seed. The seed can be dried and powdered.

Althaea officinalis

Family: Malvaceae

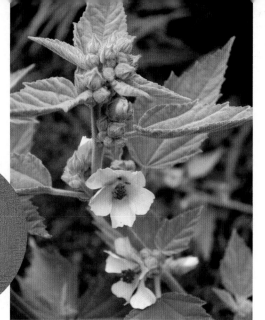

Roast the roots with your veggies and use the leaves in salads.

Marshmallow

Modern marshmallows (made with sugar or high-fructose corn syrup, gelatin, and flour) bear no resemblance to the original confections, which were made from the root of this plant, soaked in cold water to release a soothing mucilage and then pounded and sweetened with sugar or honey. Certainly it was a lot more healthful than the modern version! It was later revised to become a royal European dessert—a spongy mix of sugar, egg whites, and ground marshmallow root.

Description

This perennial plant, with its grayish green, soft, wavy, arrowhead-shaped leaves and pink, saucer-shaped flowers, holds quite a bit of thick mucilage in all of its parts, especially the root. It's a close relative of hollyhock (the root of which can be substituted for marshmallow root, in a pinch), and generally takes a slim, tall form, waving gracefully in the slightest breeze.

Preparations and Dosage

Marshmallow root can be made into tea decoctions, tinctures, syrups, capsules, and tablets. You can also use the leaves to make teas or tinctures during the growing season, when the root isn't available (although their action is somewhat milder and their mucilage level is lower).

Make a cold-water infusion, and let it steep for 30 minutes. Strain out the root, and drink 1 cup of the tea several times daily.

Healing Properties

Marshmallow root reduces irritation and inflammation and is especially favored in herb formulas and products, or even taken by itself, to treat urinary and respiratory tract infections and bowel irritation and inflammation.

Marshmallow tea is very soothing and has a mild anti-inflammatory action. Herbalists recommend it to ease the symptoms of a sore throat, cystitis, stomach irritation, ulcers, and diarrhea. Externally, it is used as a poultice to soothe skin irritation. The root contains up to 35 percent mucilage, which forms a soothing gel that coats, cools, and moisturizes wounded, inflamed tissue.

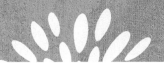

Safety

Because it forms a thick gel, strong marshmallow tea may theoretically interfere with or delay the absorption of some pharmaceuticals. If you are taking such medications, wait about an hour before taking marshmallow.

In the Garden

This graceful, herbaceous, marsh-dwelling plant does equally well in full sun or shade, as long as it gets enough water. You can even place it in a boggy spot, keeping in mind that the most mucilage is produced in deep, fertile, sandy loam soil that has good drainage. A half wine barrel or similar size pot works well for container growing. If you plant marshmallow in the ground, though, be aware that it's highly sought after by gophers, so if you have these pests, surround the root with a gopher cage. Voles can cause problems in the eastern United States, though this problem can be solved by trapping them or adopting a good feline hunter! Since the plants are tall and can be floppy, they make a lovely showing when grouped together; space them about 10 inches apart. The seed will germinate in the early spring with a little help from stratification, and you can also divide the root to propagate plants.

Harvesting Marshmallow:

You can collect up to 10 inches of the topmost stems, or several leaves, ideally when the plant is in flower. After the second year of growth, the root can be harvested at any time, but the mucilage concentration will be highest in the fall—and the older the plant, the more chance that the root will become pithy, dry, and less useful. Cut the root into small, uniform pieces to dry. It reabsorbs water easily, and insects will be very attracted to it, so store it in a tightly sealed container.

Verbascum spp.

Family:
Scrophulariaceae

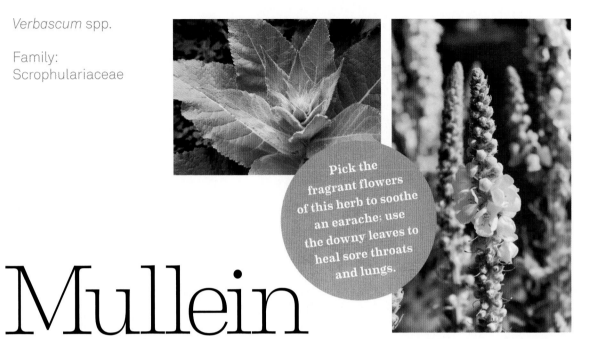

Pick the fragrant flowers of this herb to soothe an earache; use the downy leaves to heal sore throats and lungs.

Mullein

Though originally from Europe, mullein has gone wild in North America, growing in every state and province. You'll find it singly along roadsides and in large patches in fields. Herb gardens wouldn't be the same without it—from flower to root, it's full of medicine that can be used in very diverse applications. Smoking mixtures from several cultures include it to soothe the lungs, and the flowering stalks were once coated in wax or oil and used in place of torches, supposedly by witches during their midnight rituals. That's why one of its ancient names is "hag's tapers."

Description

This stately biennial has long, soft, hairy, lance-shaped or oval leaves that take a basal rosette shape the first year and appear all along the flowering stalk the second year, becoming smaller as they ascend. The flowering stalks can reach 8 feet tall, and the plant can be 3 feet wide. The flowers are round, yellow, about 1 inch across, and appear in midsummer to late summer.

Preparations and Dosage

Mullein leaves are usually made into infusions: Steep for 30 minutes, strain out the leaves, and drink 1 cup several times a day. Tinctures are sometimes used, but these are rather weak. To make mullein flower oil, place the fresh flowers in enough olive oil to cover, steep them for a few days, filter out the flowers, and store the oil in amber glass bottles or in a dark cupboard. Use 2 to 4 drops, depending on the age of the user, in an affected ear, morning and evening.

Healing Properties

Mullein leaves are favored in teas and other preparations for treating coughs, laryngitis, colds, excess mucus, and even bronchitis and asthma, and they're considered a tonic for the lungs. They contain soothing mucilage and anti-microbial compounds that help fight infections and have an expectorant and soothing action on the mucous membranes of the respiratory tract.

Both mullein leaves and flowers are often used as a lymphatic cleanser, which translates to better skin and immune health. Drops of the flower oil are used in the ear to reduce inflammation, earaches, and infections of the eustachian tubes, inner ear, and ear canal. The root of the plant is used in teas to ease the symptoms of urinary tract irritations or infections, as well as to benefit the prostate gland.

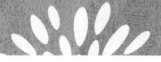

Safety

The fine hairs on the leaves can cause throat irritation if they're not completely filtered out of mullein teas. You can use an unbleached coffee filter to make sure you get them all. Contact with the hairy leaves might cause itching in sensitive individuals. Otherwise, no concerns are noted.

In the Garden

Mullein is a sturdy, self-seeding, deer-resistant biennial that will tend to choose new spots in your garden each year. We leave them in the spots they select, hoping that they'll end up in the rear, since they can achieve such height and width (and don't transplant well). They prefer full sun and poor soil and do well in an arid climate. After the second, flowering year, you can either uproot and compost the plant or, in warm climates, cut the stalk to the ground after flowering is over; it may come back as a tender perennial. In four-season climates, you can hope for reseeding. In fall or spring, sow seed directly and pack it down into the surface of the soil. The seed needs light to germinate, so don't cover it.

Harvesting Mullein: Snip off healthy leaves at any time of year. Gently pull off the open flower when the dew has dried but outside temperatures are cool. They are very fragile, so take care not to crush or bruise them, and keep them cool. If you're harvesting the root, dig it up in the fall after the first year. Chop it into small, uniform pieces to dry. The leaves take weeks to dry—you can slit them to hasten the process, but don't use high heat, as they'll discolor. The flowers don't dry well, and we don't recommend trying!

Urtica dioica

Family: Lamiaceae

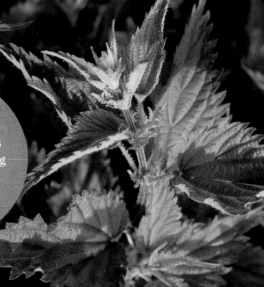

"Touch me not" without gloves, but use the leaves as a strengthening spring and summer tonic.

Nettle

Nettle's sting is so well-known it has entered the language on its own: To "nettle" someone means to irritate him or her. That sting is the result of tiny hairs filled with irritating chemicals that are released when the plant is touched. Yet when cooked, the sting disappears and nettle then becomes a most delicious and nutritious meal. This plant is found around the world and is steeped in history. It has been used for fiber, parchment, cosmetics, and food, as well as medicine. The common name probably derives from the fact that it was historically used as material for fishermen's nets.

Description

Nettle is an upright, deer-resistant perennial that grows 2 to 4 feet tall, spreading by means of creeping underground stems. The green leaves and aboveground stems are covered with stinging hairs. Clusters of greenish flowers appear at the tops of the branches and are sometimes hard to distinguish from the seeds, which follow quickly in summer's heat.

Preparations and Dosage

Concentrated nettle tea can be made by simmering the nettle tops for 30 to 60 minutes. Drink ½ to 1 cup of the tea around mealtimes, although just once a day should provide some benefits. Commercial nettle leaf tinctures can be found, but they tend to be weak. Nettle rhizome tinctures, tablets, and capsules are widely available. Follow the package directions.

Include nettle tops (harvested before flowering) in soups and casseroles, steamed like spinach. You can also use them as a mild rennet substitute for coagulating milk during cheese making.

Healing Properties

Nettle leaves are valued for their diuretic, antihistamine, anti-inflammatory, and nutritional properties. Herbalists recommend them to treat hay fever, arthritis, rheumatism, anemia, cystitis, water retention, and gout, among many other traditional uses.

Extracts of the underground stems (rhizomes) are made into capsules and tablets and are sometimes blended with saw palmetto or other herbs to reduce prostate inflammation and ease painful urination caused by an enlarged prostate. Tinctures and other preparations of nettle seed are thought to be good for the kidneys and are recommended as a general tonic and to help prevent or remove kidney stones.

For generations, midwives and many other natural-care practitioners have recommended nettle tea or concentrated extracts in capsule or tablet form as a tonic for women, even during pregnancy, to help "build the blood" (although this use has not been documented in formal clinical studies). Nettle leaf has unusually high concentrations of calcium and other minerals and is thought to be useful as a concentrated all-herbal nutritional supplement.

Safety

Beware the stinging hairs! Although arthritis sufferers report relief in the areas where nettle has stung, you might want to wear long sleeves and gloves when harvesting. Allergic reactions to the sting are common, and some people react more than others. The stinging feeling usually abates within hours or, rarely, by the next day. Drying nettle reduces the sting, and cooking eliminates it entirely. No concerns for internal use after the herb has been dried or cooked have been noted.

In the Garden

The "official" species is native to Europe and Asia, but there are species native to North America, all found near streams or lakes (and all equally medicinal). So you can guess that the plant likes partial to full shade and moist, rich soil; it also enjoys a nitrogen-rich fertilizer once a year or so. Its underground runners will spread easily under these conditions. Take care to place nettles away from the borders of beds where unsuspecting visitors might brush against it. Sow the seed on the surface of the soil and cold-stratify it, or start seedlings in the fall for cool winter conditioning. Or, better yet, dig up rhizomes in the fall, cut them into 6-inch pieces, and replant them horizontally.

Harvesting Nettle: First off, wear sturdy gloves and thick clothing. Take the top 6 to 12 inches of the fleshy, flexible stem with the leaves, and then strip off and include healthy leaves from the lower, woodier portion of the stem. If you harvest early enough in the season, you can cut the plant down to the ground after harvesting and you'll get fresh growth and a second harvest. Don't use the leaves after the seed has matured, as they develop oxalate crystals, which are irritating to the kidneys if used long-term. Harvest the rhizome in the fall or winter, after the herb has died back, starting in the second year. Harvest the seeds when they are mature but not brown. Leaves and seeds dry easily, but the rhizome should be sliced or chopped into pieces for drying.

Origanum vulgare

Family: Lamiaceae

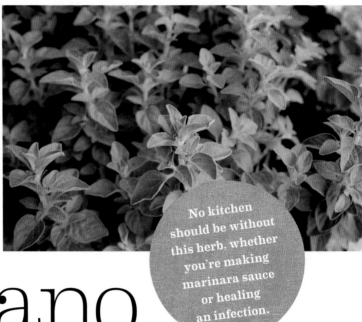

No kitchen should be without this herb, whether you're making marinara sauce or healing an infection.

Oregano

Could we be about to suggest that pizza is actually a healthy meal? We won't go that far, but read on, and plant some oregano right away! Research has confirmed that oregano oil is one of the strongest antibacterial and antifungal agents available. The word *oregano* means "joy of the mountains," a tribute to its sparkling flowers and flowing habit in its native Mediterranean habitat.

Description

This herbaceous perennial has branching stems that can trail as long as 2 to 3 feet and flowers that range from white to pink in an egg- or globe-shaped spike. There are many varieties and hybrids, and the round leaves may vary in size, hairiness, and color, ranging from green to grayish. You'll marvel at the swarms of bees, butterflies, and other pollinators around the flowers in summer. Marjoram (*O. marjorana*) differs in its slightly sweeter fragrance and the absence of strong thymol and phenol content (the antibacterial constituents). Thyme contains the same active chemicals and can be used similarly.

Preparations and Dosage

Make a standard tea and drink several cups daily after meals, or add 1 to 2 droppersful of tincture to hot water or tea. Take the powdered herb or oil in capsules, following the directions on the label. Or you can make your own oil and use it in cooking or massage it into your feet or hands to efficiently absorb its benefits. You can also add a drop of purchased essential oil to 1 ounce of olive or almond oil and use that in the same way.

Healing Properties

The volatile fraction of the herb (the component that is released when it's heated) contains high amounts of the terpene thymol, one of the most potent, broad-spectrum antimicrobial chemicals found in plants. Many studies have shown its effectiveness against a variety of pathogenic organisms, including listeria and MRSA (methicillin-resistant *Staphylococcus aureus*) bacteria.

Oregano is a common ingredient in cooking sauces, and you will get some of the antioxidant benefits by ingesting it that way. It can also be used to treat upper respiratory tract infections and for stimulating digestion (although you'll want to use more concentrated forms such as the infusion, tincture, oil, or freshly dried herb in capsules). Many other properties have been ascribed to the herb over the centuries, including sedative, calming, antiseptic, and pain-relieving actions. You can also find the essential oil, diluted with olive oil, in capsules, or you can make your own oil, and take it to prevent intestinal parasites. Oregano oil acts as a mild herbal antibiotic (compared with pharmaceuticals) to treat all manner of mild infections, including respiratory and urinary tract infections.

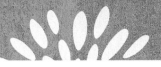

Safety

Do not take the essential oil internally unless it's in very small doses (1 to 3 drops) or the internal use has been recommended by a trained health professional. When used as an addition to food or in tincture form, oregano has no reported safety issues.

In the Garden

Deer-resistant oregano loves full sun and dryish soil that's well-drained and limey. It spreads easily by layering and seed drop, and in temperate climates it will pop up in unexpected places. It is easy to start by seed, stem cuttings, layering, or digging up a spreading mass and taking a portion of the roots and stems. Marjoram and oregano are both Mediterranean in origin and are not very cold hardy, although this differs among cultivars. If you're not gardening in a warm climate, you might need to grow it as an annual. Indoors or out, it will spill nicely over the edge of a pot if given a warm, sunny location.

Harvesting Oregano: For cooking, use just the tender leaves and add them near the end of the cooking process so their medicinal benefits will be preserved. You can include the flexible stem along with the leaves in your herbal preparations, and when the plant has flowered and is declining, you can cut it to the ground, water and fertilize it with a little fish emulsion or compost, and wait for another fresh green flush to emerge. To dry oregano, just make sure it isn't exposed to sunlight or high heat; the end product should look green and vibrant, just like the plant itself.

Mahonia aquifolium

Family: Berberidaceae

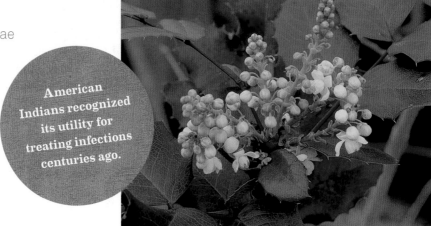

American Indians recognized its utility for treating infections centuries ago.

Oregon grape

Not many of us can cultivate the great Native American remedy goldenseal (*Hydrastis canadensis*) because of its need for shady hardwood forests and deep, rich soil. Goldenseal root is one of the most important berberine-containing herbal agents—famous for its antimicrobial action—but deer-resistant Oregon grape is a maintenance-free substitute for goldenseal that is available in standard nurseries, and nearly all parts of the plant can be used.

Description

This spiny, shrubby evergreen perennial's bright yellow button flowers and sour blue berries make it a very attractive plant to have around. Its glossy, holly-shaped leaves are unmistakable, whether the variety you find is the small *M. repens* or the larger *M. aquifolium*, which grows to 3 to 5 feet wide and tall. The yellow stems and roots are bitter tasting.

Preparations and Dosage

Make a standard decoction of the roots or lower stems and drink ¼ to ½ cup several times daily. Oregon grape root is often combined with cleansing herbs like burdock, dandelion, or red clover to regulate the liver and bile, according to traditional herbal practices.

Oregon grape root and other berberine-containing herbs, such as coptis (*Coptis chinensis*) and goldenseal, and even a purified extract of berberine itself, can be found in commercial formulas and purchased online. Follow the label directions for these products. Tincture products are also available, and compresses of the tea can be placed on boils, acne, and areas of skin irritation.

Healing Properties

The roots and lower stems of Oregon grape contain the yellow alkaloid berberine, which has broad-spectrum antibiotic activity and has been recently studied for its ability to reduce inflammation in the body, regulate blood sugar, increase insulin sensitivity, and lower cholesterol.

Oregon grape root is associated with the liver and gallbladder, having a cooling, or inflammation-reducing, effect on the liver and a regulating action on the bile. Berberine-containing herbs like goldenseal and the Chinese herb *huang lian* or coptis are used worldwide to help relieve inflammatory conditions of the lower abdominal area (especially those associated with the intestines) and liver (which also benefits gallbladder inflammation). Oregon grape root tea, tincture, and other kinds of extracts are especially indicated for skin problems such as dermatitis, eczema, boils, and acne, and they have a beneficial effect on gastric ulcers, as well.

Safety

Any herb with berberine is contraindicated during pregnancy because reports show that it can lead to neonatal jaundice. However, despite claims to the contrary, berberine does not have an abortifacient action. Nonetheless, don't use berberine-containing herbs during pregnancy and lactation without the advice of a qualified health practitioner or doctor.

For the most part, berberine-containing herbs like Oregon grape root are very safe. Don't exceed the recommended dose or use it for more than 1 or 2 weeks without advice from an herbalist. Berberine can lead to as much as a 50 percent increase in blood levels of some pharmaceuticals.

In the Garden

Native to—guess where?—and extending throughout the higher altitudes of the Pacific Northwest and into Canada, Oregon grape will adapt to sun or partial shade and is cold hardy throughout much of the continental United States. It likes rich, moist, mildly acidic, well-drained soil but will tolerate poor drainage. In the right conditions, it will spread by runners. Don't worry if its leaves become bright red after several years of growth; that's typical. You can prune the plant back in spring to shape it if it gets rangy, but don't prune too severely. Most people take cuttings or try root division with its stolons because propagating from seed is difficult. If you want to try, you should sow seed in the fall or cold stratify it for 3 months for seeding in the spring, and even then germination will be erratic.

Harvesting Oregon Grape:

Dig the root during the dormant season (you can try replanting the crowns) after 2 or 3 years. Thankfully, there is an alternative that avoids destroying the plant: You can collect the stems, discarding the upper portions that have no yellow color, and the berries. Cut the roots or stems into small, uniform pieces for drying.

Mentha × piperita and
M. spicata

Family: Lamiaceae

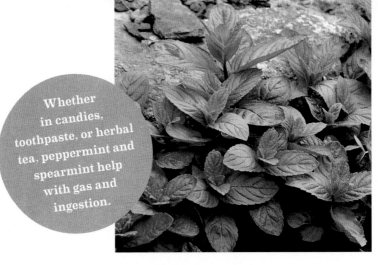

Whether in candies, toothpaste, or herbal tea, peppermint and spearmint help with gas and ingestion.

Peppermint *and* Spearmint

In one version of the several myths surrounding her, the Greek nymph Menthe was turned into a plant by her father, a river god. What auspicious beginnings! The cool scent of mint blesses everything from candies and desserts to toothpastes and cleansers. This is a plant that plays rampantly throughout the garden and has successfully interbred and crossed throughout history, resulting in countless hybrids and cultivars.

Description

Mints are perennial and herbaceous. Both peppermint and spearmint spread easily by runners and have distinctive, unique aromas. Peppermint's leaves are often smaller and darker and the stems more purple than spearmint's, while spearmint has leaves that are more textured and a lighter green. Peppermint has a flowing, sprawling habit, while spearmint tends to grow in a more upright fashion.

Preparations and Dosage

You can make infusions, tinctures, syrups, and creams with both peppermint and spearmint. And you can sprinkle the oil on potpourris for its aromatherapeutic benefits. Drink a cup of your infusion after meals as desired. A small bottle of peppermint oil is a good thing to carry with you if you are prone to gas or digestive upset after meals; just add 2 or 3 drops to a cup of hot water. You can prepare your own versions of many of the commercially available body-care products containing peppermint oil, including cosmetics, oral care formulations, and throat lozenges.

Healing Properties

Peppermint is one herbal tea that can be found in nearly every mainstream restaurant. Why has it persisted? Maybe because the flavor is so familiar and refreshing and the tea so effective at preventing and relieving gas after a meal.

Make a strong infusion of peppermint tea, 1 quart at a time, and keep it in the refrigerator. (It will keep for up to a week.) Warm it up a cup at a time during the cooler months and drink it cool or even iced during the warmer months. It is relaxing to the intestinal tract and relieves gas pains, nausea, vomiting, heartburn, morning sickness, and the crampy symptoms associated with irritable bowel syndrome and colitis. Peppermint tea is frequently indicated for easing unpleasant symptoms associated with the common cold, flu, fevers, and headaches. It's soothing to the stomach and helps stop hiccups, burping, and heartburn. Spearmint has many of the same beneficial actions, but it is much milder.

Safety

Peppermint tea is safe to use in moderation during pregnancy and nursing. When you make the tea, don't steep it for too long (more than 30 minutes) because this increases the tannin content, which could irritate your stomach, though that is unlikely except in cases of very high doses.

The safety of menthol, one of the main active ingredients in peppermint, has been questioned in the past. However, no studies have shown evidence that menthol can produce an irregular heart rhythm. The essential oil should be used sparingly, in 1- to 3-drop doses. Keep in mind that mint candies marketed as "curiously strong" contain a fair amount of peppermint oil—with no warning.

In the Garden

All mints do well in full sun to partial shade and like rich, moist, alkaline soil. They don't do well in extreme cold or extreme heat. Water them well and regularly in hot weather, preferably with drip rather than overhead irrigation, and give them a fertilizer that's high in nitrogen, such as manure, to increase the plants' oil production. They are great candidates for container growing because they will spread aggressively in your garden, and if they're in the ground, you may want to limit the spread of their roots by planting seedlings in large, bottomless cans sunk into the soil. Mints don't reproduce reliably from seed, so take stem or root cuttings, layer them, or tease out a small section of an existing patch.

Harvesting Peppermint and Spearmint:
Snip the top 6 to 9 inches of lush growth before the plants reach full bloom, and then cut the remainder to the ground for another flush of growth. Keep your harvest cool and in the shade until you get indoors. Follow the same rule when drying mints: Make sure the herb stays in darkness, and avoid high heat. Because of the high volatile oil content, mints have a short shelf life. Like basil, mints can be frozen in resealable plastic bags and thawed for later use.

Trifolium pratense

Family: Fabaceae

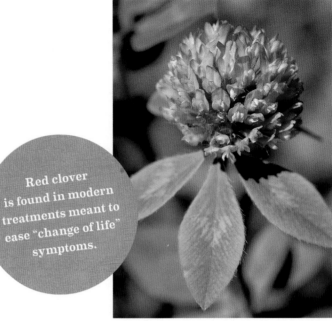

Red clover is found in modern treatments meant to ease "change of life" symptoms.

Red clover

This all-around wellness herb and blood purifier is a key ingredient in herbal blends popularized during the early 1900s and used in cancer treatment, including Essiac, Dr. Christopher's Red Clover Combination, and the Hoxsey formula. Red clover has been an Old World symbol for luck and abundance since ancient times. And when it arrived in America with the early colonists, its use quickly spread among American Indian tribes.

Description

This stout clover has deep pink—not red—plump, round flowerheads that each contain numerous, small, pea-type flowers above a three-leaved bract. The leaves are marked with a single pale chevron. The lax stems trail up to 2 feet, creating a soft green mass.

Preparations and Dosage

Make a strong infusion or tincture of red clover tops, and drink $\frac{1}{2}$ to 1 cup two or three times daily. Commercially available red clover preparations include tinctures and concentrated and often standardized extracts (containing consistent amounts of genistein) in capsules and tablets, as well as syrups and elixirs. Follow the package instructions.

Healing Properties

Red clover flowering tops are a veritable pharmacy, containing many active compounds that reduce inflammation, activate your immune response, and improve liver function. According to traditional medicine, preparations of this herb are effective expectorants, regulate blood flow, and help your body heal skin problems such as eczema, psoriasis, acne, and dermatitis.

Red clover formulas are known as "blood purifiers," which is likely due to their active chemicals—flavonoids and other compounds known as phenolics—which act as antioxidants, have anti-inflammatory properties and mild estrogenlike activity, and are stimulating to the liver and bile. Blood purifiers are thought to slowly alter the function of cells and tissues to bring them closer to a normal, healthy function. They are also thought to help create a healthy inner environment for the wellness of your skin, your body's largest organ. Red clover is a component of many formulas recommended by herbalists to help the body eliminate toxins and fight cancer.

Red clover contains isoflavonoids like genistein, which has been widely studied and is sold in dietary supplements as a natural estrogen alternative.

Safety

Red clover can be used regularly as a moderately strong tea infusion. Avoid taking it during pregnancy because of its alleged estrogenic effect. Theoretically, red clover preparations may potentiate, or strengthen, the effects of anticoagulant drugs. However, the coumarins in red clover are not like pharmaceutical anticoagulants (such as dicoumarol or warfarin), but are much milder in their action.

In the Garden

Red clover grows wild in open meadows and pastures. (The species name, *pratense*, means "of the meadows.") It loves full sun and rich, fertile, well-drained soil—but it's not picky. Water it regularly until the plants look big and healthy, and then let it go dry between waterings; this mild drought stress will bring on the flowers. Red clover is a short-lived perennial, but in most areas you'll sow it yearly. Treat the seed with inoculant or stratify it, and direct sow in the fall (if you don't get a snowy winter where you live) or very early spring.

Harvesting Red Clover: When the blossoms are open and vibrant, pick them by holding them gently and snapping them off with your thumbnail. You can include the triad of leaves just below the flowerhead. They will brown as they mature, but as long as the browning is less than one-third of the flower, they are still medicinally strong. Collect clover early in the day, when there is only light dew, to help preserve the color. Keep harvesting every 2 or 3 days to keep the flowers coming. They dry quickly, so keep a close eye on them to avoid overdrying them. Before you store them, press the centers of the flowers to make sure there's no moisture left. Store in a cool, dark place to keep the color from fading.

Rhodiola rosea

Family: Crassulaceae

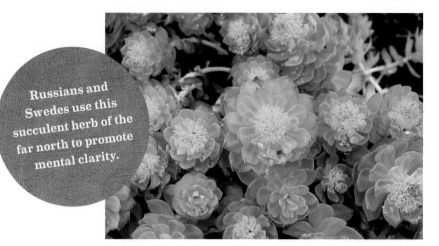

Russians and Swedes use this succulent herb of the far north to promote mental clarity.

Rhodiola

If you live at high altitudes or have a short summer, this is the plant for you. It has a long history of use in Tibet and mountainous countries throughout Eurasia, especially Scandinavia and Russia, and was known to ancient Greek physicians and Chinese emperors. In Siberia, newly married couples have traditionally received rhodiola to aid fertility. Its natural populations in northern countries are threatened because of the high worldwide demand for this plant—which is a perfect reason to grow your own.

Description

This perennial succulent is a low-growing, dramatic, 4- to 10-inch beauty with several green rosettes at its base. Fleshy leaves spiral around the flowering stems that shoot up, and star-shaped yellow flowers cluster at the top. The dried root is lightly rose scented. It's found growing wild at high elevations, but it can be coaxed to grow lower.

Preparations and Dosage

Make a tea from chopped rhodiola root and steep it for a few hours. Sip ¼ cup two or three times a day. (You can add a little licorice to improve its flavor.) Or make a tincture with a 70/30 menstruum (70 percent alcohol to 30 percent water), and take ¼ to ½ teaspoon in a little tea or water two or three times daily.

Standardized extracts of the root (guaranteed to contain 3 to 5 percent rosavins and 1 percent salidroside, the active constituents of the plant) are commonly sold commercially, and most of the clinical studies conducted were performed with a few widely available products. Clinical trials that showed positive effects studied doses of at least 340 milligrams and up to 680 milligrams per day, taken for 3 to 6 days before the effects were felt.

Healing Properties

Rhodiola is immensely popular in Scandinavia and Russia, and its popularity is increasing in many other countries, including the United States and Canada. The root is considered to be an important adaptogen (a substance that helps your body adapt to stress and restores its normal, healthy function) and is used to help counteract stress and fatigue and promote physical vitality and good mental functioning.

The root of rhodiola is likened to ginseng in Scandinavia and has many beneficial properties ascribed to it, including use as an antidepressant, antioxidant, antiviral, immune system stimulant, nervine, heart and lung tonic, and much more. More than 20 clinical studies (some of them small, preliminary, and uncontrolled) show that the regular use of supplements containing rhodiola has beneficial effects including improving memory, counteracting mental and physical fatigue, and improving mental and physical performance, especially after mental work or physical exercise. At least two studies show measurable reductions in anxiety and nervousness with rhodiola use.

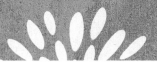

Safety

No known interactions with other herbs or drugs have been recorded.

In the Garden

Rhodiola prefers dry, sandy soil and tolerates cold like the arctic plant it is. Place it in full sun in the rock garden and don't mulch or fertilize it. Try experimenting: It's known to grow in a variety of soils and is fairly adaptable. It may even self-seed if it is in a suitable site. Make sure it has excellent drainage if you have rainy, wet winters.

Starting from seed is easy if you soak it overnight and sow on the surface of the soil in fall, winter, or very early spring, when the soil will remain cold for a few weeks or months and moisture levels will be low. You can take cuttings from the plant before it flowers, but the easiest propagation method is plant division. When you do this, make sure you separate off new shoots (found at the base of the plant) that have plenty of underground stem, and pot those. Grow male (red-flowering) and female (yellow-flowering) plants together if you want to save your own seed.

Harvesting Rhodiola: Dig the root after 4 or 5 years of growth. Notice how the top of the root begins to change color and connects with the base of the stems: This is the crown. You can cut the root away from this portion and replant it. Wash the harvested roots well with a strong spray of water, since they typically trap and hold grit. Chop them into small, uniform-size pieces for drying and enjoy the floral scent of the drying root!

Rosmarinus officinalis

Family: Lamiaceae

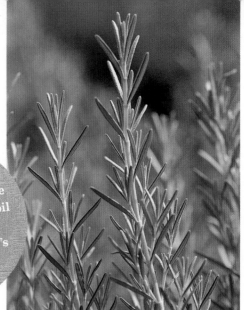

Rosemary is the herb of choice for flavoring olive oil and helping to relieve your body's aches.

Rosemary

Rosemary, the herb of remembrance, is a most versatile herb. Flavor foods and oils with it, use it to rinse your hair, scent your bath with it— you can even use it to improve your test scores! Rosemary is one of nature's best antioxidants and preservatives and is even used in the food industry. In addition to that, it is a remarkable "habitat plant" (one that attracts beneficial pollinators to the garden) and those blue flowers are often busy with bees. You should not be without it.

Description

Deer-resistant rosemary is a resinous, aromatic, woody shrub with narrow, needlelike leaves and, in original or wild varieties, delicate blue or violet flowers. (The time of bloom varies in different climates.) In nurseries you'll find dozens of varieties with widely different habits and flower colors. Some upright varieties can grow to 6 feet tall.

Preparations and Dosage

Make a tea or, for more antioxidant power, make a decoction. (This will be a stronger, more bitter blend for the hardy.) Rosemary makes a good tincture, and 1 or 2 droppersful can be added to water or tea. A teaspoon of rosemary vinegar in a little water before meals is a refreshing pick-me-up. Rosemary extract is added to many dietary supplements and foods for its antioxidant and other health benefits.

Make rosemary oil and apply it to your feet, especially between your toes, before bedtime. This medicinal application will increase circulation, reducing foot pain and fatigue after a long day of use.

Healing Properties

You may know rosemary as a culinary herb but not as an herbal medicine. Well, think again! Its chemistry is complex, including many phenolic compounds (a class of antioxidant chemicals found in grapes, pomegranates, and green tea) with powerful protective actions. Adding it to your diet on a regular basis, even supplementing daily, will let you reap the well-known anti-aging and protective effects of the antioxidants it contains.

Rosemary has been known throughout history to invigorate the nervous system and brain function, reduce fatigue, help alleviate headaches, strengthen digestive function, and benefit the cardiovascular system. In particular, its connection to the health of the heart and cardiovascular system is ancient. That makes sense, considering rosemary's powerful antioxidant and protective properties, along with the beneficial effects it has on circulation.

Speaking of circulation, rosemary has a long reputation for helping to regulate menstrual flow and ease cramping pain. In traditional Chinese medicine, pain anywhere in the body is thought to result from the stagnation of blood and vital energy, so it follows that rosemary relieves pain as it invigorates the circulation of energy and blood throughout the body.

Shakespeare wrote, "Rosemary, that's for remembrance," a saying that every herbalist knows. It refers to this herb's long-standing tradition as a beneficial memory herb.

Safety

Rosemary is both a culinary and a medicinal herb, so its safety is well established. People with sensitive skin might develop mild skin irritation if the strong oil is directly applied without first diluting it in olive or almond oil.

In the Garden

We often say that all rosemary really needs is sun—shade will result in insipid, lackluster growth. Around the Mediterranean Sea, you'll find it hanging on cliffs and chalky hills. It likes sandy, rocky, poor soil and excellent drainage. Water it lightly as it is getting established, and never water it again. If you live where winters are mild, prune it down to the first green growth yearly, or it will become woody. If your winters are severe, grow it in pots and take it inside each year before the ground freezes. Choose a spot indoors that is sunny but not too warm, and mist the plants every week or so. Make cuttings, layer, or divide the roots to start new plants.

Harvesting Rosemary: Harvest the tips of the branches (as long as the stems are flexible and are not longer than about 12 inches) or the leaves stripped from their stems at any time of year. The oil content of the leaves is highest when the plant is in flower. Dry it at low heat and in darkness; this one browns easily.

Salvia officinalis

Family: Lamiaceae

The sage in your spice rack is the one you want—out of 500 members in the genus *Salvia!*

Sage

Sage is a favorite garden plant and culinary herb. The Latin name *Salvia* means "to save," which gives us a clue as to its position of honor in the herbal pantheon: This is an ancient, sacred herb. The garden sage that is such a familiar seasoning is only one of the many species in the genus; there are many other cultivars and varieties. But its best uses far outstrip its popularity as a stuffing ingredient for the Thanksgiving turkey.

Description

Sage is only one of several medicinal salvias. It is a grey-green, woody, shrubby perennial with purple, pink, or white flowers and textured leaves, and its aroma is unique. Deer-resistant garden sage grows to about 2 feet high and 2 to 3 feet wide, providing a safe haven for myriads of pollinators.

Preparations and Dosage

Make a standard infusion of sage and drink $1/2$ to 1 cup two or three times a day. Because sage contains small amounts of thujone, a strong compound, it's wise to avoid drinking more than this quantity for more than a few weeks. Take a break of a week or two before resuming. As a mouthwash, or for the throat, gargle a strong infusion two to five times a day, as needed.

Healing Properties

Sage, as a tea, is the first herb we recommend for reducing the pain and discomfort of a sore throat. During cold season, we often carry a small bag of tender sage leaves and chew on them, swallowing the healing and anesthetic juice to numb the unpleasant soreness and help speed healing. Sage-lemon tea is an excellent drink for treating colds and flu, especially if you add some thyme for extra antibacterial action.

Sage is also famous as an herbal deodorant, and you'll find it in commercial sprays and creams. This use make sense, considering sage's known antibacterial action and pleasant, earthy scent.

Nursing mothers traditionally used sage to help dry up the last flow of milk. A mild infusion of the herb has been used for this purpose, but we recommend avoiding the herb altogether when pregnant or nursing because of the possibility that infants could be sensitive to thujone, one of sage's compounds. At the other end of the childbearing years, herbalists recommend sage for reducing the sweating associated with menopausal hot flashes.

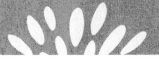

Safety

We don't recommend using sage tincture or oil internally because they both contain much higher amounts of the terpene thujone than does the tea. Sage is not appropriate for continuous, long-term use, and the herb should be avoided during pregnancy and nursing.

In the Garden

Sage is happy in full sun and cool to hot temperatures, as long as the soil is dry or at least well-drained. It's a great candidate for a rock garden. We've found that it can succumb to wilt, especially if it gets too much water, and therefore can be short-lived. It will not often survive a prolonged freeze, although you can give it extra protection by covering it with leaves, straw, or another light mulch. If you live in a severe climate, you might want to play it safe and grow sage in a protected spot or even in a pot, so you can bring it inside during the winter months. Pinch sage back (to keep it from flowering) regularly during the growing season, and then trim it back by one-third or more during each dormant season. In those severe winter areas, don't prune sage back until the new growth starts to emerge in the spring.

You can start it from seed (which will be easier if you stratify it), or you can take cuttings in the spring before the plant flowers. Layering also works well when the stems are long and lanky with spring growth.

Harvesting Sage: You can harvest the leaves, before the plant flowers and through the full flowering stage, including any flexible stem. Don't harvest when the leaves are wet, and for the highest essential oil content, wait until midday. You can encourage new growth by pruning sage down to its first green growth during the heat of the summer season. Dry sage leaves in complete darkness and at a steady low temperature to help prevent browning.

Prunella vulgaris

Family: Lamiaceae

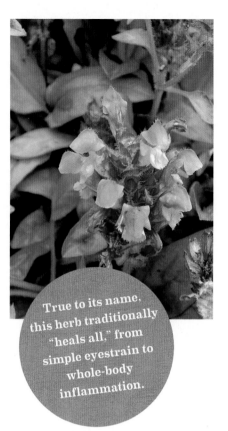

Self-heal, heal all

True to its name, this herb traditionally "heals all," from simple eyestrain to whole-body inflammation.

You'd think a plant with a name as auspicious as this one would be dramatic and imposing. Instead, it camouflages itself in your lawn. But it has been used internally and externally since at least the 2nd century in both China and Europe. Its botanical name, *Prunella,* derives from the German word *brunella,* which comes from *die Braune,* meaning quinsy (a throat abscess), for which it was commonly used in the Middle Ages.

Description

Self-heal is a creeping perennial that volunteers in moist places like woods, pastures, subalpine meadows, and, of course, lawns. It sends up a flexible, branching, flowering stalk that can reach 1 foot tall, with soft oval or lance-shaped leaves and beautiful pink to blue-violet flowers on spikes.

Preparations and Dosage

Self-heal is used as a tea, in tinctures, and as an extract in capsule and tablet form. Make a strong infusion, and drink 1 to 3 cups a day. For the tincture, use 1 to 2 droppersful in warm water or tea two to four times daily. Follow the label instructions on other products.

Healing Properties

Self-heal is a great example of an herb that is used both in traditional Chinese and Western cultures. In Europe, the herb has been used since the Middle Ages and is mentioned in 16th-century herbals as a wound-healing herb and a gargle for diseases of the mouth and tongue.

In China, self-heal has been used since at least the 14th century as a cleansing herb that normalizes liver enzyme output and reduces fevers. In traditional Chinese medical thinking, each internal organ associates with a sense organ, and the liver is associated with the eyes. Thus self-heal tea can be used as either a wash or a tea to help ease eyestrain, red and itchy eyes, sties, and other eye inflammation. The tea or extract can also help relieve dizziness and headaches when these symptoms are associated with a liver imbalance.

Self-heal is loaded with protective and antioxidant compounds known as phenolics, which act as antioxidants and have anti-inflammatory properties similar to the ones found in pomegranates and green tea. Since the taste is mild and refreshing, the herbal tea or extract can be used regularly as a healthy, calming drink for the liver, the skin, and the whole body.

A number of current studies show that self-heal can protect the blood vessels and has antiviral effects against influenza, herpes sores, and HIV/AIDS.

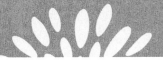

Safety

No concerns are known.

In the Garden

Self-heal will want to be placed in partial shade; you can grow it in full sun, but it will need ample water. Give it fairly moist soil, and don't fertilize it too much. Once the flowerheads have turned brown, cut them back to the ground to encourage another bloom. Self-heal is low and spreading and can die back during dry summers. It's somewhat frost tolerant, and though it's often a short-lived perennial, it reseeds and spreads easily by runners. Self-heal is a very pretty groundcover, weaving in and around other plants, and it also looks lovely cascading over the edge of a pot.

The seed sows best after cold stratification, or you can start it early in spring, before the last frost. Cuttings have a low success rate, but dividing the plant is nearly always successful.

Harvesting Self-Heal: Gather the flowering tops and any additional leaves below the flowering tops. In Western medicine, we consider the flowers to be potent as long as at least one-third of the head is blooming and no more than one-quarter is browning. In traditional Chinese medicine, however, the flowers are gathered when they are "wilting," meaning already brown. Make sure this herb is dried at low heat, since it degrades quickly.

Scutellaria lateriflora

Family: Lamiaceae

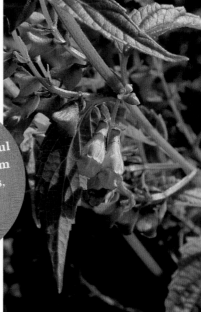

The leaves and stems of this beautiful herb are used to calm nerves, ease stress, and reduce anxiety levels.

Skullcap

For today's fast-paced, stressful urban lifestyles, you can't beat the soothing, nourishing properties of skullcap. American Indians used it long before European settlers did, and on the other side of the globe the Chinese used a related species, *S. barbata.* Both that Chinese skullcap and another, *S. baicalensis* (primarily harvested for its root), are making their way into Western herbal use and can be grown in much the same way as *S. lateriflora.*

Description

This hardy herbaceous perennial is native to eastern North America and has a delicate profile, growing to almost 2 feet tall. The leaves are green and mintlike (without the minty smell), and the flowers are small and sky blue to purplish. The helmet-shaped flower inspired the plant's common name, and each seed looks like a "little shield," which is the meaning of the Latin genus name, *Scutellaria.*

Preparations and Dosage

Take skullcap as a standard tea or tincture. The flavor is slightly bitter, so it acts as a relaxing digestive tonic. We recommend adding more flavorful digestive herbs, such as orange peel (which also has relaxing properties).

Healing Properties

Skullcap is widely recommended by herbalists as a nervine, which in the broadest sense is an herb that has a tonic effect on the nervous system. Skullcap is used to reduce nervousness and anxiety and in some cases to treat insomnia, and modern studies have confirmed these uses. It is mild, and not a true sedative. But if it's taken for some weeks it can reliably help to calm jittery nerves, and it works well with a stronger herb, such as valerian. Skullcap's action complements other nervines, and it is useful in a larger group, such as with hops, passionflower, and lavender.

Skullcap is also used for spasms, neuralgia, and epilepsy. In earlier times, the herb was often prescribed as a cure for rabies and the bites of mad dogs. Naturally we're hoping you'll never have to use it that way! Other older folk uses include treating excessive sexual desire (monks used to drink the tea to maintain their pious demeanor, although there is no modern evidence to support this use or the idea that the herb has an antitestosterone effect) and to relieve addictions.

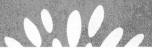

Safety

Skullcap is considered safe to use for the long-term, as well as during pregnancy and nursing. One caveat, though: In commercial preparations, skullcap is sometimes adulterated, or germander herb from the genus *Teucrium* is substituted for it. Germander is stressful on the livers of sensitive individuals and is best avoided. To ensure that you really have the correct herb, which is entirely safe, grow your own!

In the Garden

Skullcap is native to riverbanks and damp areas and wants to receive ample water. You can plant it in full sun to partial or afternoon shade, depending on the amount of moisture and heat it will get. Fertilize it once or twice a year, and weed it often to eliminate competition around the delicate seedlings. Because its profile is not dense, a close grouping has a nicer effect than single plants placed around the garden will. A cluster in a large pot also works well.

Skullcap starts easily from seed but can take a while to germinate. Start it outdoors in the fall, stratify and start it indoors in the spring, or direct-sow it in cool soil. Cuttings and root divisions are less successful.

Harvesting Skullcap: Collect the top flexible stems and leaves, from early flower through the late flowering stage. If you cut it back to the ground early in the season, you'll get a second flush of growth. The leaves dry quickly, but the stems take quite a bit longer.

Stevia rebaudiana

Family: Asteraceae

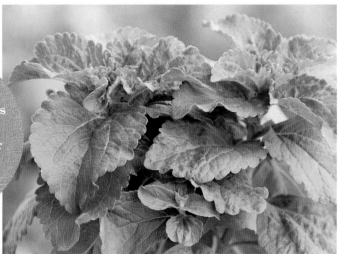

This herb is used to flavor Diet Coke in Japan and is now a best-selling natural sweetener in the United States.

Stevia, sweet leaf

Stevia is an amazing traditional noncaloric sweetener. The active compounds are up to 300 times sweeter than table sugar, but stevia does not cause tooth decay or raise blood sugar levels. In the face of the diabetes epidemic, it's time to take a good look at this beautiful plant!

Description

Native to tropical regions of Paraguay and traditionally used to sweeten maté tea (a popular South American caffeinated drink), this tender shrub has scalloped green leaves and tiny white flowers, and it grows to 2 feet tall. In warm, humid climates the leaves will be almost 2 inches long, but they're much smaller if the plant grows in cooler conditions or if it's stressed.

Preparations and Dosage

Add stevia leaves—fresh, dried, liquid-extracted, or powdered—to recipes in which you use sugar or other sweeteners. Follow recipe guidelines and don't be afraid to experiment; however, in large doses, stevia can be overpowering and have an unpleasant undertone. Some people describe its aftertaste as licoricelike and sometimes slightly bitter (although you'll now find products with very little aftertaste). Make a tincture from your own plants with a menstruum of 25 percent ethanol (you can use 50-proof vodka), and keep it in 1- or 2-ounce dropper bottles that you can bring with you to sweeten drinks and foods. Of course you can also finely powder your own dried leaves or make a dried extract.

Healing Properties

In the United States, stevia is used almost exclusively to sweeten foods and drinks. But unlike sugar, stevia extracts have some "side benefits" (as opposed to "side effects"). It does not raise or lower blood sugar or blood pressure, and it has been shown to actually inhibit tooth decay. It has no calories and is fairly stable in cooking. It also aids digestion and settles the stomach.

In parts of South America, stevia was and still is traditionally recommended to treat hypertension, for use as a diuretic and cardiotonic (strengthening the heart muscle), for preventing cavities, and even to fight fatigue, depression, and infections. Some recent American studies have shown that it is able to significantly reduce blood pressure and improve quality of life. Other studies, including those focused on type 1 and 2 diabetes, blood pressure, blood glucose, and glycated hemoglobin tests (a measure of possible diabetes) have shown more mixed results.

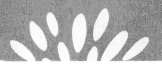

Safety

Fairly large clinical trials have uncovered no tolerability or safety issues. Stevia has been used in the food industry to flavor drinks for many years, particularly in Japan and South America. Many studies on stevia's safety have been published, and after initial confusion and misregulation in the 1990s, it is now classified as GRAS (generally recognized as safe) by the FDA.

In the Garden

If you don't live in the tropics, this yummy plant will be an annual for you. It's the perfect herb for a sunny windowsill or bright porch. Outside, it will also need full sun, moist but not soggy soil, and good drainage. Give it some fertilizer and make sure that it is grown in rich soil. Stevia loves humidity, so it grows well in a greenhouse and will appreciate occasional misting wherever you place it. Grow it in a pot on the deck and take it indoors in the winter, unless you live in a completely frost-free area.

Starting stevia from seed can be frustrating: The seed will only mature during long, humid growing seasons, and germination rates are very low. If you try this method, be sure to keep the seed on the surface of the soil, just pressing it in, and keep it consistently moist. You'll have more success with stem cuttings and root divisions.

Harvesting Stevia: Only use the leaves, since the stems will have a slightly stronger taste and edge toward bitterness. For best results, snip the leaves before the plant flowers. If you're harvesting them outdoors, be sure to keep the harvest in the shade. While drying, maintain a low, steady heat to avoid browning.

Hypericum perforatum

Family: Hyperiaceae

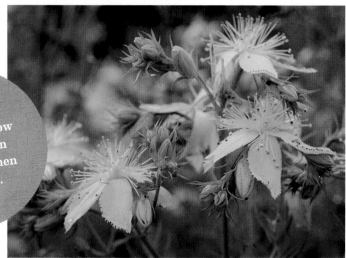

This herb's glorious yellow flowers turn blood red when squeezed.

St. John's wort

So named because it was traditionally gathered on St. John's Day (June 24), when the plant is typically in full bloom, St. John's wort travelled from Europe to the United States, where it promptly got into hot water with ranchers because it causes photosensitivity in cattle that graze on it. What a pity that as a result it has been declared a noxious weed in some areas; while it is invasive, it is also a sacred herb of the sun from ancient times and an important and popular healing plant today.

Description

St. John's wort is an upright perennial that grows to 3 feet tall and has bright yellow flower clusters at the ends of its stems. Its small, elliptical leaves are dotted with translucent spots—hence its species name, which refers to the perforations. It thrives in disturbed soil (places where native vegetation has been removed and the soil is bare) in open, sunny spots. The plant forms a wide, low, green, spreading mat in the winter.

Preparations and Dosage

Homemade tinctures and the infused oil are easy to make and are widely used. For the tincture, take 2 to 3 droppersful in a little water or juice twice daily. The oil can be applied liberally.

Standardized and nonstandardized, or full-spectrum, extracts are available in capsule and tablet form. Follow the label instructions on commercial products. The dose can be adjusted according to the size and sensitivity of the user, with smaller or more-sensitive people taking 900 milligrams a day and larger or less-sensitive people taking up to 1,800 milligrams.

Healing Properties

Public awareness of this plant bloomed in the mid-1990s when newspaper articles proclaimed that St. John's wort had the same positive effect on mood that Prozac does, but without the side effects. Since then, much has been written about it, and it has arguably been the subject of more clinical studies and meta-analyses than almost any other natural medication. It's amazing that St. John's wort was known as a magical plant and was recommended for anxiety 2,000 years ago. Those ancient uses eventually led to the modern discovery of its antidepressive effects.

Herbal clinicians today recommend the flowering tops to treat mild to moderate depression and insomnia; to relieve chronic nerve pain such as peripheral neuropathy, shingles, and trauma; and to treat external injuries involving nerve damage. St. John's wort is sometimes prescribed for children who wet the bed. Externally, the infused oil is widely touted for reducing skin inflammation and the pain of scrapes, burns, sunburns, bruises, and strains.

Safety

Consult with a physician or experienced herbalist before using therapeutic doses of St. John's wort for the long-term. Avoid regular use when taking life-sparing pharmaceuticals such as anti-rejection drugs, blood-thinners, and antiretroviral drugs, as this herb can lead to changes in blood-serum levels of these medications. Photo-sensitization is possible, but it will probably only occur in fair-skinned individuals who are using large and regular doses.

In the Garden

St. John's wort loves full sun, dry conditions, poor to average chalky soil, and a nice cold winter. It spreads by runners and easily self-sows in favorable conditions. In fact, it's considered invasive and is illegal to cultivate in California, Colorado, Montana, Nevada, Oregon, Washington, and Wyoming. If you don't live in any of these states, you can start it from seed: Stratify it and press it into the surface of the soil. You can also try dividing the plant, but we've had far less success with that method, as it doesn't transplant well.

Harvesting St. John's Wort:
Skim off the flowering tops (the top 1 to 4 inches) when part of the inflorescence is in flower and the rest is going to seed. If you're harvesting a large amount, don't pile it up thickly because it holds field heat and bruises easily. You can wear gloves or wash your hands afterward to guard against excessive absorption of the hypericin in the plant. The flowering tops dry quickly, but their shelf life can be shorter than the normal guideline of 1 year, and sometimes as little as 6 months. Be sure to store them in a cool, dark, and dry location.

Thymus vulgaris

Family: Lamiaceae

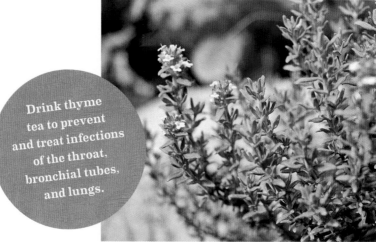

Drink thyme tea to prevent and treat infections of the throat, bronchial tubes, and lungs.

Thyme

Thyme is one of several exemplary medicinal herbs that also double as mouth-watering culinary accents. It is a beautiful edging plant, and it offers so much strong antiseptic action that no garden should be without it. You may find yourself asking, Does anybody really know what thyme it is? The answer may surprise you: At least 350 species worldwide make it a very large and interesting group of plants, and all of them have healing properties.

Description

Thyme is a delightfully aromatic, low-growing perennial shrub that's often woody. Depending on the variety, it is sometimes erect and sometimes a groundcover, forming dense mats. Its flowers range from white to ruby red, and its leaves are tiny. Bees love thyme, as do chefs and herbalists. You'll find many mouthwatering varieties with exciting scents and flavors, but for the most medicinal potency, use plain old English thyme.

Preparations and Dosage

A mild to medium-strength tea is our favorite way to use this herb. Infuse the fresh or dried flowering tops and leaves, and increase the percentage of herb a bit from our standard tea infusion formulation to make a fairly strong tea. Add a little honey or licorice tea and drink ½ to 1 cup frequently throughout the day as needed. To preserve the tea for use outside the home, add a little 25 percent (50 proof) alcohol and ½ teaspoon of vitamin C powder to it. You can store this mixture in the refrigerator for at least a week. Thyme is also available in tinctures, lozenges, syrups, sprays, and cold and flu preparations of all kinds. Follow the label directions.

Healing Properties

Thyme tea is a classic healing drink known in European culture as the medicine of choice for uncomplicated upper respiratory tract infections—colds, flu, bronchitis, and strep throat. Drinking 1 or 2 cups of the tea daily when you're warding off an infection is a smart idea. Thyme is also recommended for improving digestion, coughs, and mucus congestion, and it's used externally as an antimicrobial wash.

In the Garden

Thyme enjoys full sun and well-drained soil—its roots will rot if it's overwatered or if it experiences a lot of rain without having good drainage. Many varieties are hardy in four-season areas, but they prefer a Mediterranean climate with hot, dry summers and mild winters. Prune back about half the length of the growth in spring—or down to the very first growth on the stems by the time the herb flowers—and then again severely in fall (warm climates) or very early spring (four-season climates) to keep the plant from becoming woody. Seeds often have low germination rates and are prone to damping off, so many growers prefer to take cuttings or divide the plants in the spring.

Harvesting Thyme: Just before bloom or while it is in bloom, clip the leaves and stems just above the woody portion of the plant. Dry the entire stems, and then rub or strip the leaves off for storage.

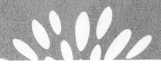

Safety

There are no concerns for thyme tea or preparations, with the exception of the volatile oil, which is quite irritating to the skin and mucous membranes. To use the volatile oil, always dilute it in an equal amount of olive or almond oil. The tea is perfectly safe to consume during pregnancy.

Curcuma longa

Family: Zingiberaceae

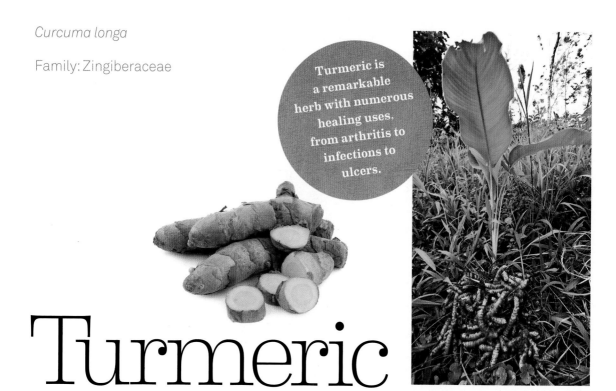

Turmeric is a remarkable herb with numerous healing uses, from arthritis to infections to ulcers.

Turmeric

Turmeric was used by the Assyrians more than 2,500 years ago. It is sacred to the Hindu faith and is an all-star in the kitchen as well as the medicine cabinet. In fact, turmeric is an herbal poster child for the "functional foods" movement, demonstrating that foods and spice extracts can help prevent chronic disease when used regularly at mealtimes and in supplement form. That bright yellow color in curry dishes? You guessed it!

Description

Turmeric is a large-leaved, slim plant that grows 2 to 5 feet tall and has a round stalk and a yellow flower that doesn't always appear in cultivation. It originates in moist, tropical forests of the Indian subcontinent. The brownish yellow root is the part that's used medicinally.

Preparations and Dosage

You won't be surprised to hear that we recommend cooking with turmeric! You can add it liberally to foods, consuming the equivalent of ¼ to ½ ounce (7 to 15 grams) per day. Teas and tinctures are also quite effective. Make a standard decoction with other herbs such as ginger, and drink ½ to 1 cup twice daily. Both the extract of turmeric rhizome and the isolated constituent curcumin can be found in many herbal and dietary supplements. For these commercial products, follow the label directions. You can also make your own salves to apply externally.

Healing Properties

Turmeric is a priceless treasure in the herbal kingdom, both as a spice that colors and flavors dishes throughout Asia and as a modern medical superstar. It burst upon the scene with healing anti-inflammatory gifts at just the moment when medical science was realizing that most, if not all, chronic diseases are driven by underlying inflammatory processes in the body—what the ancient and modern Chinese medical sages call "yin deficiency."

The root of turmeric contains the strong anti-inflammatory substance curcumin, which acts with other compounds through several biochemical pathways. Traditionally, the spice was used in teas and extracts to treat arthritis, tendonitis, heart conditions, and liver and digestive problems. Now preliminary clinical studies confirm its use for cancer prevention and the treatment of precancerous lesions, painful digestion, and stomach ulcers. Externally, turmeric is applied to wounds and bites and is used for preventing and treating infections.

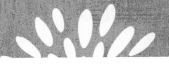

Safety

There are no safety concerns when using turmeric in cooking or teas, but do avoid using the concentrated or standardized extract during pregnancy. Fijian women use turmeric to increase production of mother's milk, but it can have an antifertility effect when taken in very high doses, as is possible with standardized extracts. Also, use caution with the standardized extract if you are taking blood thinners. Very high doses of concentrated extracts of turmeric have proven to be toxic in some animal tests, but lower doses have not.

In the Garden

Unless you live in the tropics, you'll have to grow turmeric in a greenhouse or on a sunporch. Start with purchased rhizomes and place them in moist, rich soil with good drainage in dappled shade (or full sun, if you're in the far north). You can even buy a fresh root at the market and place it in a pot at home. To multiply your fresh pharmacy, cut the rhizome into pieces, making sure each one contains at least one eye (the wrinkled protuberances on the root itself). Place the pieces a couple of inches into the rich potting mix, with the eyes pointing up, and make sure the soil stays moist and warm. Shoots will form in 2 to 3 weeks. If you want the turmeric to remain in the pot for a while, make sure you place it in one that's deep enough to contain the root, which grows 8 to 10 inches long. Turmeric will not survive if temperatures around it drop below about 60°F, and consistent direct sun will scorch the leaves. Ginger loves the same conditions and is cultivated in a similar manner, so you can enjoy them together!

Harvesting Turmeric: You will want to wait until your plant is at least 1 to 2 feet tall and well established before you harvest it when it dies back in the winter. If you've planted in springtime, your plant will wither and droop when cold weather arrives. Lift the root from the soil, and remove the crown, replanting both the crown and small pieces of the root, if you like. Chop turmeric into small, uniform pieces to dry, and store it in a cool, dark place. You can powder the root for cooking.

Valeriana officinalis

Family: Valerinaceae

Need help falling asleep or staying asleep? Herbalists recommend valerian above all other herbs.

Valerian

One of valerian's early names was *Phu*, and some say this is because of the sound you might make when you smell the root! Old, dry valerian has a reputation for smelling like dirty socks. But fresh roots have an exotic and enticing scent, and certain species were used as perfume in Tibet and were said to be attractive to the opposite sex. Don't let the odor be a hindrance to exploring this well-studied and traditionally used sleep and relaxation herb, or to including it in your garden. It is so beautiful and easy to grow. Your cat will love it, too, and may nearly destroy the plant, just like catnip.

Description

This lovely, hardy perennial has pleasantly scented roots (when fresh), deeply cut leaves, and tall, flowering stalks capped with small white or pink flowers in lacy, spraying clusters. Garden valerian (*V. officinalis*) is the species traditionally used for healing.

Preparations and Dosage

In our experience, the strongest and best preparation is a tincture of the freshly harvested and washed roots. Make it fresh every year (or at most, every 2 years) to maintain effectiveness. Take ½ to 1 teaspoon (and up to 1 tablespoon, if needed) of the liquid tincture in a little water or tea. (Chamomile tea is a good choice.) For chronic insomnia, take the tincture morning and evening for a week or longer; valerian develops a stronger effect with consistent use.

Dried products in capsules and tablets are not as calming or effective as extracts made from the fresh root. The active compounds in valerian are rather unstable when exposed to light and oxygen, so the least-effective way to use the root is to dry and powder it.

Healing Properties

If we wanted to give you a sound bite, we'd say that valerian is "the sleep herb." Certainly it's been the most important herb for at least 10 centuries in European herbalism and culture to calm the nervous system and promote healthy sleep. In one interesting clinical study, two groups of volunteers were outfitted with motion sensors and recorders attached to their wrists. One group was given a valerian preparation and the other was given a placebo pill. The next morning, researchers found that the people in the valerian group fell asleep faster and tossed and turned significantly less than those in the placebo group.

Valerian preparations are recommended by herbalists for insomnia, anxiety, nervous tension, and emotional upset, as well as for related conditions like nervous digestion and headaches. Other uses include relieving menstrual cramps, reducing heart palpitations (when blended with hawthorn or hops), and treating pain (when combined with chamomile).

Safety

Some people have reported experiencing an unexpected stimulating effect after taking valerian root extracts. This is much more likely to happen when the product is prepared from old, dry roots and is unlikely with a fresh preparation. Large doses have sometimes been reported to cause headaches, but this appears to be a rare, idiosyncratic effect. Depending on the strength of the tincture and the sensitivity of the individual, an effective dose for one person might be excessive for another. Don't exceed the recommended dose without professional advice.

In the Garden

Valerian is native to moist forest margins, marshes, and edges of fields, so it will enjoy full sun but will also tolerate partial shade. It does need moist, rich, loamy soil (and can even tolerate poorly drained areas), so in very hot climates you'll want to lean toward shadier spots. Give it compost or other organic fertilizer regularly. Some commercial growers remove the flowering stalk to strengthen the root, but we can't bring ourselves to cut down that gorgeous example of botanical expression! It will self-seed and spread under favorable conditions.

You can start valerian from seed or by root division. The seed is short lived, so plant within 1 year after you receive it, and sow it in cool temperatures on the surface of the soil. Be sure to keep it moist until germination.

Harvesting Valerian: Dig the root after the second or third year of growth, after the plant dies back in the fall and before it fully leafs out in the spring. You may want to pinch the flowering tops back to encourage better root development. You'll have to wash valerian roots really well: They hold dirt and grit tenaciously. Chop the roots into small, uniform pieces for drying. Did we mention that they have quite a noticeable aroma? Be sure to store the dried root away from heat and light.

Vitex agnus-castus

Family: Lamiaceae

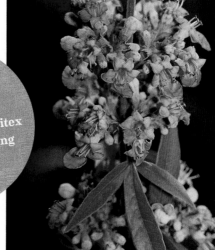

Long valued as an herb for treating female health concerns, vitex is useful for easing symptoms of PMS.

Vitex

Even though it's sometimes considered a classic "women's herb," the Renaissance name for vitex fruits was "monk's pepper," so called for their ability to decrease the libido of the abbey's residents when sprinkled on their food. Since they probably needed it often, the monks no doubt had the "habit" of carrying it, well, in their habits! Herbalists and medical researchers alike now believe that vitex has the ability to regulate the reproductive hormones, so it has acquired a reputation as a true hormonal tonic.

Description

This lovely deciduous shrub, which has been known since ancient times, can grow to be a small tree in hot climates. It is cultivated as an ornamental in the Mediterranean and elsewhere. Vitex has distinctive, aromatic leaves that are divided into lance-shaped leaflets, and in summer it bears abundant purple or lavender flowers on spikes. The flowers are followed by small reddish to brownish burgundy berries in the fall, but these only develop where the growing season is long and warm.

Preparations and Dosage

Make a tincture of the aromatic fruits (the berries) in strong alcohol (150-proof or stronger vodka). Take 1 to 2 droppersful in the morning around breakfast, or for a stronger effect, try 1 to 2 droppersful at night. Avoid taking more than 4 to 5 droppersful a day. We recommend only making and using *tinctures* with vitex: Teas are not the best way to prepare this herb because the active compounds are not particularly water soluble, and the tea is not delicious by any means. For commercial products, including standardized extracts, follow the label instructions.

Healing Properties

Aside from the Chinese herb *dang gui* (*Angelica sinensis*), vitex is *the* classic female herb and is often recommended by herbalists for relieving unpleasant symptoms of PMS. Clinical studies verify its ability to relieve cramps, breast tenderness, and mood swings associated with the menstrual cycle, even when compared with conventional pharmaceuticals. In addition, vitex is certainly worth a try as a first treatment before taking one of the SSRIs (selective serotonin reuptake inhibitors, primarily known as antidepressant medications, such as Paxil, Prozac, and Zoloft) or other drugs, because the side effects are minimal.

Vitex extracts are known to act through the stimulation of the pituitary gland to regulate a number of important sex hormones, including progesterone, which it increases. Imbalances of these hormones have been clinically associated with symptoms of PMS, such as breast tenderness. Other symptoms for which vitex is recommended include irregular or excessive menstruation, late periods, spotting, uterine fibroids, and even hot flashes, though studies are not very conclusive in regard to the latter. The tincture is also recommended for relieving acne in teenagers, with variable success.

Safety

The side effects of vitex are minimal, based on a number of clinical trials and long traditional use. Both research and clinical experience show that regular use of vitex might interfere with the effectiveness of birth control pills. Don't take it if you are using a progesterone supplement, and avoid its use during pregnancy.

In the Garden

This Mediterranean plant needs full sun and well-drained soil. It tolerates both drought and heat, but it's also hardy to -10°F and can withstand windy locations. However, if you're in a four-season climate, it may not flower or bear fruit. Try to give it the sunniest, warmest site you can. And don't fertilize this one: Rich soil results in pale flowers. If you want to keep the plant small and bushy, prune it back in late winter. It's a great deer-resistant addition to your garden.

You can start vitex from seed if you scarify, stratify, and/or soak it in warm water and then sow it on the surface of the soil without covering it. But taking cuttings from spring and early summer growth is the easiest way to propagate this plant.

Harvesting Vitex: You can use the leaves in cooking and in spice blends, and some people use them medicinally, as well. But we recommended harvesting the berries for your herbal remedies. Pick them in the fall, when they turn from tan to a purplish color and separate easily from the stems. Make sure you harvest them before autumn rains and cold weather cause them to mold or blacken on the tree. Separate the berries from the stems before you dry them rather than after.

Artemisia absinthium

Family: Asteraceae

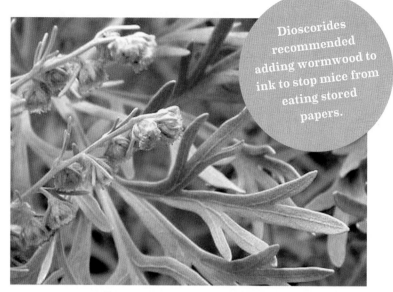

Wormwood

This distinctive, lacy shrub is best known in some circles as the main ingredient in the legendary liqueur absinthe, and it is certainly one of the most bitter herbs you can grow. Just remember the herbalists' adage, "Bitter to the taste is sweet to the stomach," and think of wormwood as a trusted ally if you need a good remedy when you overindulge in food or drink.

Description

This lanky, alternately upright or horizontal perennial is a very common ornamental, widely grown for its ease of care and beauty. Wormwood has profuse, silvery, gray-green, feathery leaves and tiny yellowish flowers, and it is pleasantly aromatic. It can expand to almost 3 feet high and wide and tends to sprawl and become woody at the base.

Preparations and Dosage

Make a standard infusion, and drink ½ to 1 cup of the tea before a meal once or twice daily. A typical daily dosage is 3 to 6 grams of the dried tops or leaves. We do not recommend using wormwood in tincture form.

Wormwood oil is a major ingredient in the famous mind-altering drink absinthe, but the sale of this beverage is controlled today in most European countries and in the United States because it contains the toxic constituent thujone.

Healing Properties

Wormwood is a time-honored herb for treating intestinal parasites, as its name implies. This aromatic shrub was known to the ancients and has a very long history as a bitter herb added to magical elixirs and liqueurs created in monasteries throughout the Middle Ages from plants grown in the monks' own herb gardens. Even today, wormwood tea is widely consumed as a refreshingly bitter digestive tonic to counteract pain, gas, abdominal distension, and upset stomach after a rich meal or overeating. It is helpful for treating loss of appetite, difficulty with fat digestion, and gallbladder complaints.

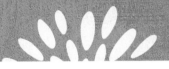

Safety

Avoid wormwood during pregnancy and while nursing, and be careful that you don't exceed the recommended dosage or use it for more than a few weeks at a time. Some herbalists warn to avoid wormwood in any form if you have hyperacidity (for instance, if you experience frequent heartburn). Use extra caution with the alcoholic extract or essential oil.

In the Garden

Wormwood originated in open, grassy areas and on hot, dry, rocky slopes, so it likes full sun and lean, light, well-drained soil. (It is somewhat susceptible to fungus if its drainage is not good.) It is drought tolerant and deer resistant. You'll want to cut it back severely (to 6 to 12 inches) in winter to ensure healthy regrowth. Mulch or cover the plant where winters are severe. It can get rangy, so give it plenty of room in your garden. Start new plants from seed, cuttings, or root divisions. (This is a good idea every 3 years or so, as the plant can become quite woody and contorted with age.) The seed will need to be stratified and only pressed into the surface of the soil, since it germinates best with light.

Harvesting Wormwood: When the plant is in early to full flower, cut the top 4 to 6 inches of leaf and flexible stem and any leaves further down the stem. Wormwood dries easily, but it tends to clump and mat. It's easier to separate out any unusable material after it has dried.

Achillea millefolium

Family: Asteraceae

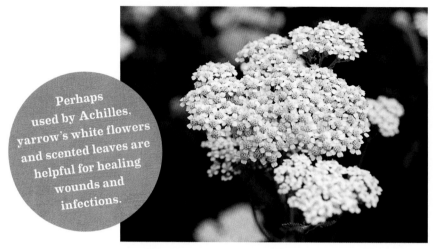

Perhaps used by Achilles, yarrow's white flowers and scented leaves are helpful for healing wounds and infections.

Yarrow

It's said that, as a baby, the great Greek warrior Achilles was dipped in yarrow by his mother, to give him his superhuman strength—but that she held him by his heel. That being the only area not covered, he was of course later slain by an arrow to his "Achilles' heel," his only weak spot. And don't forget the medieval teaching that yarrow grew in churchyards as a reproach to the dead who need not have died had they eaten their yarrow! In China, it is believed that even the stalks are powerful; they have been historically used to cast the *I Ching*.

Description

Yarrow grows as a low, spreading mat of finely dissected, aromatic leaves that reach about 1 foot high. Umbrella-shaped clusters of tiny white flowers appear above the foliage in summer on stalks up to 2 feet high. *Achillea* is native to the entire northern hemisphere (North America and northern Eurasia). If you want to grow the most potent medicine, stick to the white-flowered species and don't choose any of the other lovely flower colors that are available in nurseries.

Preparations and Dosage

Make an infusion by steeping ¼ cup of the dried flowers in 2 cups of water for 20 to 30 minutes. Drink 1 cup of the tea two or three times daily. This is a mild herb, and it can be taken regularly for 2 to 3 weeks.

A traditional combination for easing fevers and other symptoms of flu is one part yarrow leaf or flower, one part elder flower, and one part peppermint leaf. Infuse the herb combination for 30 minutes and drink it throughout the day as desired.

The leaf is well known for its ability to stop bleeding when applied directly to a wound, and you can carry it dried and powdered in your first aid kit.

Healing Properties

Yarrow tea is slightly bitter and aromatic and is a famous European remedy used to ease the symptoms of colds, flus, painful digestion, "liver stagnation" (weak bile flow) accompanied by poor fat digestion, and a feeling of fullness after meals, especially fatty ones. Laboratory studies have definitively established that yarrow has anti-inflammatory, antispasmodic (relaxing the smooth muscles found in the uterus and digestive tract), antifever, and antiviral effects. As an extra bonus, yarrow seems to have a calming effect, which can help with PMS and other nervous conditions, and it stops bleeding when applied to a wound.

It turns out that there is a fair amount of variation in the chemistry and biological actions in wild yarrow populations, so we recommend growing your own from seed or from plants obtained from one of our recommended sources rather than purchasing plants from nurseries or gathering them from wild populations.

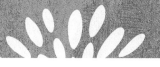

Safety

Avoid yarrow during pregnancy and while nursing unless you're under the guidance of an experienced herbal practitioner. Allergic reactions to members of the Asteraceae family, though rare, are known in sensitive individuals. They can manifest as a skin rash (even from just handling the herb, which is more likely with the fresh plant), digestive upset, or headaches.

In the Garden

Yarrow is found from sea level to above the timberline in the wild, so you know it is highly adaptable. It thrives in full sun but can tolerate partial shade, loves water but can endure mild drought, is winter hardy, and spreads quickly in cultivated (or disturbed) soil. It does like poor, acidic conditions, so don't fertilize it. Let it dry out between waterings.

You can grow yarrow from seed if you sow in the fall or stratify the seed before planting. (It's often sown directly.) But root division is another good method and can help control the plant, since it has a tendency to spread.

Harvesting Yarrow: Snip off the flower cluster when it's in full white bloom (no colored varieties, please), and then cut the stalk all the way to the ground to encourage further blooming. You can harvest the leaf at any time of year. For drying, you can also cut long flowering stalks and use the hang method, snipping the flowers off later. Keep the whole flower clusters intact when you store them.

Anemopsis californica

Family: Saururaceae

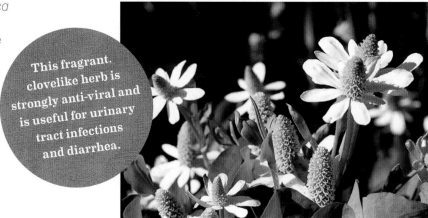

This fragrant, clovelike herb is strongly anti-viral and is useful for urinary tract infections and diarrhea.

Yerba mansa

The name "yerba mansa" comes from the Spanish colonizers of the southwestern United States and means "herb of the Mansos." In the 16th and 17th centuries, the nomadic Manso Indians lived along the Rio Grande in New Mexico. They were peaceful people when the Spanish came, and they took to Christianity, sometimes working in the missions. It was the Manso who introduced the strong healing powers of yerba mansa to the missionaries.

Description

Yerba mansa is a low-growing, herbaceous perennial with soft, fleshy leaves that develop characteristic red spots as they age. It bears spiky, cone-shaped white flowers that rise dramatically above the basal structure in the summer. The underground stems (rhizomes) and roots have a spicy, pleasant aroma and ginger-clove–like flavor, and the creeping stolons reach out and extend the patch in moist environments. Yerba mansa is found in seasonally wet or boggy areas in deserts all throughout the Southwest. The plant slowly reddens as the season progresses, until fall frosts send it underground for the winter.

Preparations and Dosage

Make a tea from the rhizomes and roots by simmering them for a few minutes, then steeping for 20 to 30 minutes. Drink ½ to 1 cup at a time, two or three times daily. The tincture can also be used, and the fresh or dried herb is sometimes added to remedies for colds and flu or digestive problems in capsule or tablet form. You can powder the dried rhizome and herb and pack it into capsules yourself. Take 2 capsules, three times daily, around mealtimes. The tincture and the capsules are likely to have the highest anticancer activity.

Healing Properties

Yerba mansa is widely respected today as an antiviral and decongestant herb for treating respiratory tract infections such as colds and flu. The Eclectic physicians, early 20th-century medical practitioners, cited it especially for "a full, stuffy sensation in the head and throat, [especially] whenever we have cough with expectoration," according to Finley Ellingwood, MD, author of the influential 1919 book *American Materia Medica, Therapeutics and Pharmacognosy*. They also recommended the herb for urinary tract troubles and diarrhea, and as a gargle to be used frequently throughout the day to help treat swollen gums and sore throats. The tea tastes great, and the plant is easy to grow and beautiful in the garden, to boot—what else could one ask for? No human studies have been performed with the herb, but laboratory studies show that it has antimicrobial and anticancer activity, specifically against breast cancer.

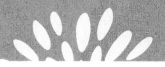

Safety

There are no specific concerns found in the literature.

In the Garden

This striking plant is found along seeps, stream edges, and wet meadows, and it is known as a bog plant, but we've found it to be very adaptable in the garden both to consistently moist soil and to low irrigation (although if you want it to look lovely, choose the former). It also adapts to full sun or partial shade and to acidic soil, though it prefers alkaline. It will tolerate a mild freeze. It's perfect for a water garden or a nondraining barrel or decorative tub.

The seed is challenging to germinate and can take up to 3 months, though it responds to warm temperatures. It's easier to split off the running stolons and root them at the nodules (raised areas on the stems where leaves arise).

Harvesting Yerba Mansa: You can use the herb (all of the above-ground portions, when in flower), the root (anytime from fall dieback until the plant fully leafs out in spring, preferably from the third year onward), or the whole plant (anytime from leaf-break through full flower). When you dry it, separate the aboveground portions from the root, and chop the root into small, uniform pieces.

MEDICINAL WEEDS AND THEIR USES

Many weeds are maligned, but they actually have very effective healing components. Use an internet image search to verify the identities of these medicinal weeds.

COMMON NAME	LATIN NAME	PARTS TO USE	USES	NOTES
Chickweed	Stellaria media	Herb	Consume raw, or as an infusion or fresh tincture to assist in fat metabolism and constipation.	The mild, refreshing taste of this famous wild salad green makes it great for salads, soups, and garnishes.
Chicory	Cichorium intybus	Root, leaves	The root is used like dandelion root to benefit your liver and is roasted and ground as a coffee substitute.	Cook the greens in olive oil and garlic with added lemon to make a nutritious traditional Greek dish called horta.
Cleavers	Galium aparine	Herb	An infusion of the young, leggy stems and leaves is used to treat irritation of your urinary tract or to help prevent infections.	Add a sweetener or another soothing herb such as plantain leaf to make a better-tasting infusion.
Dandelion	Taraxacum officinale	Root, leaves, flowers	The flowers are fermented with sugar to make a wine that is thought to benefit the eyes; the roots are a noted liver tonic to promote good digestion and increase bile flow; the leaf tea and dried teas are herbal diuretics for cleansing programs.	Dandelion leaves are a nutritious green vegetable when young; they are high in potassium and other minerals.
Fleabane	Conyza canadensis	Leaves, flowering tops	Use it as an infusion several times a day to benefit the respiratory tract and to prevent colds.	One of the most common roadside weeds, worldwide.
Knotweed	Polygonum aviculare	Herb	Make a light decoction to soothe irritated bowels and loose stools and to cleanse the urinary tract.	This common, sprawling, weedy herb is found throughout the world and is used routinely in China.
Lamb's quarters	Chenopodium album	Herb	Makes a nutritious, mild-tasting infusion that is high in minerals.	Cook the young tops like you would spinach, or add them raw to salads.
Mallow	Malva neglecta, M. spp.	Leaves	Make a cold- or warm-water infusion and drink it throughout the day to soothe your urinary and digestive tracts.	Add the young spring greens to salads, or stir-fry them with garlic and vinegar for a healthful and nutritious green dish.
Milk thistle	Silybum marianum	Seeds	Blend the seeds in water, let them soak overnight, and then filter them out to make a seed "milk." This drink is high in essential fatty acids and, if used regularly, can benefit your liver.	Wear thick gloves when you collect the seeds from the prickly heads. Run the heads through a compost shredder or food processor to disengage seeds and winnow, then store in glass jars.
Oats	Avena sativa, A. fatua, A. barbata	Flowering "spikelets"	Use as an infusion or tincture as a tonic to calm the nerves and reduce irritability.	Strip the seeds from the grass tops when they're in the "milky" stage (when they exude a drop of milky starch when squeezed).

COMMON NAME	LATIN NAME	PARTS TO USE	USES	NOTES
Peplys/Garden spurge	*Euphorbia peplys*	Whole plant	Break the stem and apply a drop or two of the juice to warts for a few days to eliminate them.	This weed was used by the ancient Greeks; keep the irritating milk away from your eyes.
Plantain	*Plantago major, P. lanceolata*	Leaves	Make a light decoction and drink it throughout the day to soothe your digestive and urinary tracts.	Crush or blend fresh leaves with a little water and apply to cuts, wounds, burns, bites, and rashes to speed healing and reduce inflammation and pain.
Purslane	*Portulaca oleracea*	Herb	Eat it raw in salads or garnish your meals with it. It's the greatest plant source of omega-3 fatty acids and benefits digestion.	This succulent garden weed is widely collected in Europe.
Queen Anne's lace	*Daucus carota*	Seeds	Take as an infusion to promote good digestion and relieve gas and spasms.	This plant is a wild version of the domesticated carrot.
Shepherd's purse	*Capsella bursa-pastoris*	Herb	The tincture has been used for centuries to help slow excessive menstrual bleeding.	In Europe, it's also used as a heart tonic, combined with hawthorn leaf and flower tincture.
Speedwell	*Veronica americanum, V.* spp.	Herb	Make an infusion to relieve excessive mucus congestion, lower mild fevers, and benefit your liver and skin; make a salve to treat skin ailments like eczema.	It's a beautiful addition to your garden as a bedding plant, as well.
Violet	*Viola odorata*	Leaves, flower	Make a soothing infusion to promote expectoration of mucus and to soothe a sore throat and cough.	The common scented English violet has a delightfully scented flower and can spread in gardens.
Wild geranium	*Geranium carolinianum, G.* spp.	Whole plant	Make a light decoction and drink a cup several times a day to ease loose stools.	The young leaves can be eaten as a green vegetable.
Wild lettuce	*Lactuca virosa, L.* spp.	Herb	Juice the whole plant and add it to celery and carrot juice as a bitter tonic to promote good digestion.	It's a wild form of common garden lettuce, but contains a milky juice and is more bitter.
Willow herb	*Epilobium* spp.	Leaves	Make a mild-tasting infusion that is soothing to your digestive tract and treats your prostate.	This is an extremely common garden herb.
Yellow dock	*Rumex crispus*	Root, leaves	Make a root decoction or tincture to help regulate your bowels and activate the bile to help in cleansing programs.	The young spring greens are high in vitamin A and can be stir-fried or used in soups.

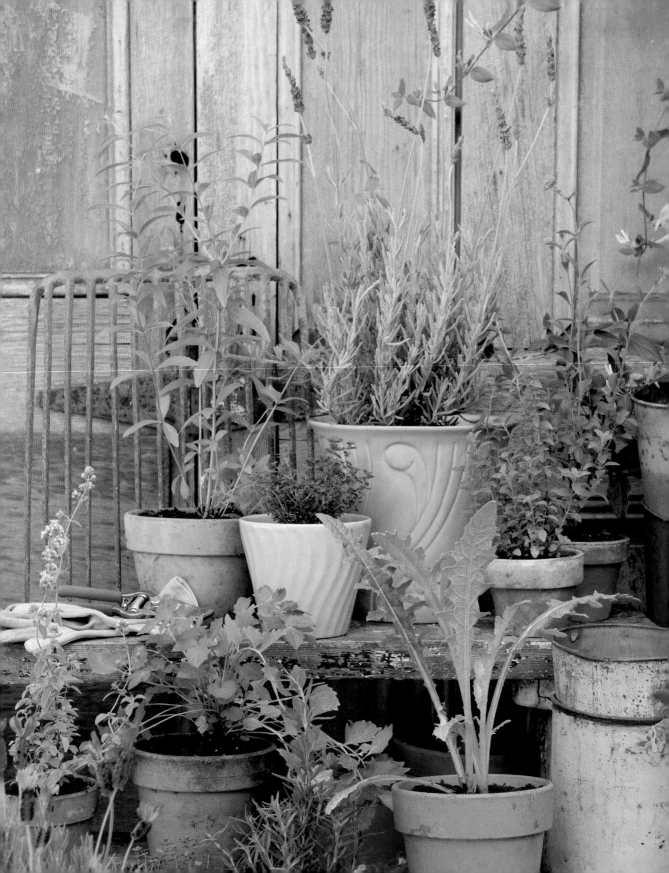

PART 2

Grow It

You don't need to be an experienced gardener to begin growing your own remedies! Learn the basics needed to plant, grow, and properly harvest herbs, as well as tips on establishing healthy soil, best habitats, and plant preferences, whether you have a traditional outdoor garden or containers indoors or out. Discover how to gather herbs, save seed, and dry and preserve your harvest to create healing remedies. By raising herbs yourself—even if you only grow a single plant—you'll have a ready source of organic and healthy medicine for harvesting and healing.

The healing garden: It conjures up images of lush landscapes that indulge your eyes, water features that soothe your ears, sun-baked golden pathways that guide your spirit, and cool breezes that make your skin tingle. Spend some time in these lovely natural settings and you'll find it's therapeutic just being among plants. Allow the green world into your sensual realm and you'll experience healing. Science shows that, of all the colors, green is the most soothing and rejuvenating as it passes through the retina of your eye. Just touching and smelling aromatic herbs brings minute quantities of the medicinal molecules into your body. We need moments and days of quiet reflection and contemplation to hear what the plants have to say to us, particularly because our increasingly fast-paced and multifaceted world disconnects us from nature.

You can be part of the world of healing herbs wherever you are. No matter how you choose to enter into this ancient form of self-care, you're taking an important step that can lead you in new directions. Some of us have land to plant a garden, some of us have a patio or deck with room for decorative pots, and some of us have a sunny windowsill or corner of a kitchen—you can grow herbs in all of these places. Starting a garden, indoors or out, allows you to connect with the soil, to nurture healing plants, and to grow your own medicines. When you grow herbs yourself, they're conveniently at hand when you need them most.

The Outdoor Garden

Whether you're an experienced farmer or completely new to the world of gardening, medicinal herbs offer a unique growing experience. In this section, you'll learn the steps you need to take to create a living herbal apothecary outside your door. If you have land to cultivate and would like to grow your own herbs, start right here.

From the Ground Up

Gardening begins with the soil; it's the "ground of our being," to borrow a phrase from German theologian and philosopher Paul Tillich. If you take care of the soil, the soil, in turn, will nourish and feed the plants you grow for healing and health.

Soil Types

An important first step in growing outdoors is to find out what kind of soil you have. Take a handful of soil from a couple different places in your yard or on your land, make sure each one is somewhat moist, squeeze it gently in your fist, and then examine it. If the soil in your hand is somewhat sticky and holds together in a ball, it is *clay* soil. This type of soil is high in nutrients but can be heavy and waterlogged. If the herb you want to grow needs good drainage, you should add sand, gravel, or organic matter to the soil to lighten the texture. But if your herb needs rich soil and moisture, clay soil may be fine.

TOOLS FOR GROWING HERBS

Gather the tools of your trade! If you're growing herbs outdoors, you'll need different tools than you will if you're growing them inside or in containers. Here's a checklist of supplies you'll need.

FOR OUTDOOR GARDENS	FOR POTTED OR WINDOWSILL GARDENS
Gloves, both rugged and thin (such as Atlas brand)	Thin gloves (such as Atlas brand)
Long-handled shovel, digging fork, weeding fork, and small trowel	Trowels, large and small
Clippers, loppers, and hand trimmers	Clippers, hand snips, and scissors
Various sizes of pots and seeding trays	Various sizes of pots, seeding trays, and decorative containers
Potting soil and seed-starting mix, horticultural sand	Potting soil and seed-starting mix, horticultural sand
Compost, aged manure, fish emulsion, and other fertilizers, such as Maxicrop seaweed products	Compost, fish emulsion, and other fertilizers, such as Maxicrop seaweed products

If your sample is grayish and gritty and falls right through your fingers, it is *sandy* soil. This soil type drains well, but it allows nutrients to wash away easily so it is considered the leanest soil. It warms up earliest in the spring so it may allow you to get a head start on the growing season. If the herb you want to grow needs rich conditions, you'll need to add amendments (such as compost, organic fertilizers, and other sources of organic matter) to improve the texture of sandy soil and boost its nutrient content.

If your sample is a rich brown color, smells sweetly earthy, and crumbles easily, it is *loam* soil. This is the ideal soil type because it holds nutrients and moisture, yet it's well aerated, so roots can easily expand and grow. Depending on the herb you are planting, you might add sand or gravel for better drainage or compost or aged manure to further enrich the soil.

Your site may have more than one type of soil, or even a combination of all three types. But no matter which you have, you should pay attention to the level of organic matter your soil contains. Check to see if the sample in your hand looks like it contains bits of dark-colored humus (organic matter, such as composted plants, tiny pieces of bark, and worm castings). If your soil is lacking humus, consider working in materials such as finely chopped leaves or compost.

pH levels

Soil's acidity or alkalinity is measured by its concentration of hydrogen ions, or pH (the **p**ower of **h**ydrogen). You can test a soil sample yourself or send it away for testing to determine its pH level. Most herbs and vegetables prefer pH levels to be in the neutral range (6.5 to 7.5), but some varieties are tolerant of more widely

The Benefits of Cover Crops

To add nutrients, especially nitrogen, to your soil, you can try planting a cover crop. Cover crops (such as rye, fava beans, and alfalfa) are also called green manures because they increase organic content, improve soil tilth, and feed earthworms and soil microorganisms, much like animal manures do. Cover crops are usually planted in late summer or fall, then cut down and tilled into the soil in the spring, several weeks before planting time, while they're at a green, tender stage. Cover cropping is often practiced on larger working farms, but it's equally useful for small gardens. While many gardeners turn over a cover crop with a rototiller, you can also chop down and bury a cover crop under a heavy layer of mulch or chopped leaves. Cover crops are most useful if you'll be planting annuals such as vegetables and culinary herbs that you start anew each year.

acid or alkaline soils. Excess acidity or alkalinity (below 5.5 or above 8) will make it difficult for a plant to take up nutrients. Sandy soils are often acidic (below 7), and chalky or limey soils are alkaline (above 7), but your local conditions play a role, too. You can buy fairly good, inexpensive testing kits at garden stores if you want to do it yourself, or you can ask your local Cooperative Extension Service about their testing services. They may perform several types of analysis, including measuring levels of organic matter and nutrients, and they will make recommendations for amending the soil to create ideal growing conditions for your plants. For example, if your soil is too acidic, you can add amendments to increase alkalinity, such as limestone, calcium, and wood ashes. If your soil is too alkaline, add sulfur, pine needles, leaf mold (composted leaves), and even highly diluted urea.

Nutrients

Plants have nutritional needs, just like we do. The three major nutrients, which are usually included in commercial fertilizers, are nitrogen (N), phosphorus (P), and potassium (K). In purchased fertilizers, you'll see them represented on the label as three numbers separated by dashes: 5-10-5 (meaning 5 percent nitrogen, 10 percent phosphorous, and 5 percent potassium). Plants need smaller amounts of other micronutrients, such as boron, calcium, copper, iron, manganese, and molybdenum, and these are often included in fertilizer mixes, too.

Nitrogen is necessary for plants to develop healthy leaves, and you can provide it in several ways. Good sources of nitrogen include compost, aged manure, blood meal, grass clippings, and fish emulsion. Cover crops, also called green manures, are another; see "The Benefits of Cover Crops" on the opposite page.

Phosphorous is important for seed, flower, and root development in plants. Good sources are bone meal, phosphate rock, compost, and fish emulsion.

Potassium (sometimes called "potash") helps develop roots and fruits and helps plants take up nutrients. Good sources of potassium include wood ashes, comfrey tea (which is also high in calcium, iron, and manganese), algae powders (such as Maxicrop), granite dust, and fish emulsion.

How do you know if a plant needs fertilizer? Even without soil test results, you can follow these simple clues: If your herb is stunted and the stems are thin and stiff, or if the leaves are small, have yellowed, or have even begun to fall off, you may need to add nitrogen (N). If your herb has leaves that are turning purple on the undersides or at the tips, or if the stems are thin and the plant is growing slowly, you may need to add phosphorus (P). If your herb begins to look "scorched" at the leaf margins or has bleached spots, the stems are weak and wilting, the leaves are curling, and the growth is stunted, you may need to add potassium (K).

We garden organically and always have. Over the years, we've experimented with various soil amendments, but we always come back to the tried-and-true, slow-acting, self-generating superstar—compost. We apply a few inches of it each year. When you feed the soil according to the needs of the herb in question, the plants will be stronger and better able to stave off disease and pest issues.

If plants show signs of nutrient deficiency, that's the time to top-dress with a few inches of compost or to water with liquid fertilizers, such as comfrey tea, algae liquid made from commercial powders, or fish emulsion and seaweed fertilizers. Start with a watering can full of liquid, follow the directions on the commercial product (if applicable), and slowly water the soil around the plant until it begins to run off or the soil appears to be saturated.

If you've performed a soil test and you know that you have nutrient deficiencies, you can work in any of the dry nutrients at the rate recommended on the label, depending on the needs of the individual herbs. Or you can simply sprinkle the powder on the soil surface, cultivate the soil to work the fertilizer deeper into the ground, and water well.

Mulch

Mulch is simply organic material that you lay on top of the soil around your plants. It can be wood or bark chips, dry leaves, straw, crushed rock, or grass clippings. Mulch provides a barrier between the soil and the air, which helps to keep moisture in the soil, and it gradually breaks down to provide organic matter to the soil. Keep in mind that different materials may have varying levels of acidity or alkalinity, and most should not come in contact with the stems or trunks of your plants. If your summers are humid (which means that fungal problems are an issue), be judicious about adding mulch, because some organic materials can introduce pathogens. Sand, gravel, and stone may be better options for you. You can also use agricultural or landscape fabric; just fasten it down with stakes and cut holes for your plants. These fabrics (and black plastic or polyethylene, which we do *not* recommend) are used as weed barriers and water conservation aids. They have their place, particularly if you live in a dry climate or need to discourage a massive preexisting population of an intractable weed or undesirable plant, such as Bermuda grass, but natural mulches usually do the job just as well.

Light

Most herbs and vegetables need 4 to 6 hours of direct sunlight a day to thrive, but this is a general guideline only. Some plants will tolerate a wide range of light exposure, and their sunlight requirements may vary in your local climate, as well. Each herb profile lists that plant's individual needs.

Water

Herbs require water to grow, but how much is enough? Growing powerful medicinal herbs is a playful dance between simulating wild conditions (giving plants the same environmental situations that they would encounter in their homeland) and providing cultivated amenities that might improve their potency and health.

Let's look at essential oil content. Many of the herbs we grow for medicine (and food) are valued for that constituent, and we might want to pay attention to what increases it. Many members of the Lamiaceae, or mint family (basil, catnip, oregano, peppermint, and thyme) come from Mediterranean climates, where summers are hot and dry and winters are

mild. They have adapted to dry conditions for much of the year. It stands to reason that, at some point, their essential oils can be diluted if they are overwatered. Yet research has shown that *some* supplemental water given to these plants increases their foliage yield and essential oil levels.

Where you, the grower, come in is in determining when you've given your plant enough water, but not too much. You'll want to remember that clay soils hold water longer, sandy soils drain faster, and gardens on sloping hillsides lose moisture (which mulch can help retain). You'll have to assess water needs based on your conditions and the season, as well as the needs of the individual plants.

If you plan to garden on a larger scale or have limited garden maintenance time, you may want to consider an automatic watering system that consists of overhead sprinklers, drip irrigation, or a combination of the two. These systems are both time- and work-savers, relatively inexpensive, and often sold in easy-to-use kit forms. Overhead watering mimics nature, of course, and we've noticed that plants in a hot, dry environment appreciate the humidity it provides. But overhead watering in the later part of the day can set up ideal conditions for fungal diseases to develop, and it also tends to waste water. Drip irrigation can deliver water where it's needed—at the roots of the plants—through a series of tubes and emitters, but the equipment can be easily damaged and requires a fair amount of maintenance. Talk with a garden center about your needs and read product reviews online to be sure that the system you're considering is a good match for your needs.

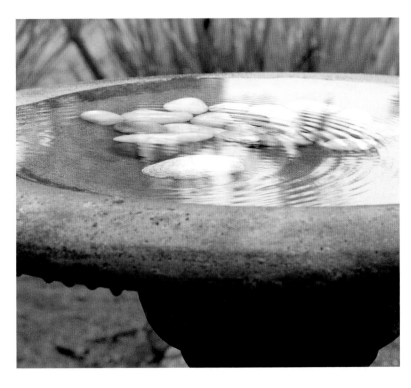

It's always a great idea to include a water feature somewhere in your garden, whether it's a pond, a birdbath, a waterfall or preformed streambed with a recirculating fountain, a Flowform (a series of connected basins that allow water to cascade in a pattern of figure eights, replicating the path water takes in undisturbed flows found in nature), a container fountain, or even a sturdy bowl sunk into the ground. A water source will attract birds and other pollinators to visit your plants and contribute to the biodiversity and function of your ecosystem.

Temperature

This element comes into play in several different ways. How do you know when to sow seeds or set plants into the ground?

First, of course, there's the temperature of the soil. Some herbs germinate best in cold soil, some in warm. Then there's timing: You'll want to learn the last frost date for your area so you'll know when you can safely plant those tender spring seedlings. (You can ask your local Cooperative Extension Service or, of course, do an online search.) Armed with this information, you'll be able to choose herbs from our recommendations wisely.

Let's Plant Herbs

Maybe you already know which herbs you'd like to grow. Take a look at the individual herb profiles and make sure the ones you're interested in growing are suitable for your region. Even if you're unsure about a particular herb, it's often worth a try. In some cases, you may be able to adjust your environment and provide comfortable growing conditions for a variety of herbs, by amending your soil and by carefully choosing planting locations for their different light and exposure conditions. Check "Plants to Grow for Herbal Healing" on page 136 to choose your plants according to their preferences for shady or sunny spots in the garden, water needs, and soil preferences.

After you make your plant selections, you'll need to decide whether to buy plants or start them from seed. See "Buying and Ordering Plants" (page 121) and "Propagation" (page 122) to help you decide.

Preparing the Bed or Row

Before you plant anything, you will want to prepare (and possibly amend, or feed) the planting area. The best time to do this is in the fall, because it allows the winter snow, rain, and wind to work their magical alchemy, along with the soil microbes and the tunneling creatures. But spring can be just as good a time for preparations, particularly if you live in a colder region.

First, clear all "weeds." (In the process, feel free to check to see if any of them appear on pages 104–105; if they do, harvest them!) Using a shovel or digging fork, break up the soil in the bed or row to a spade's depth. Next, armed with your analysis of the nutritional or textural needs of your garden, spread several inches of compost, aged manure, or fine mulch on the surface. If you know that your soil needs to be adjusted for pH level or a plant's nutritional needs, now is the time to add your

organic, slow-release fertilizers. Work them into the soil. If you know you will be growing herbs that achieve their best medicinal potency in lean soil, omit or go easy on the amendments.

If you need to loosen heavy clay soil, add compost, perlite, vermiculite, coir (shredded coconut hulls), or sand. To firm and enrich sandy, poor soil, add sterilized topsoil, compost, or aged manure.

Raised Beds

There are advantages to growing herbs in raised beds. If your drainage is poor, a raised bed will give you a lot of room for excess water to drain away from plant roots. If you have a tired back or use a wheelchair or are otherwise differently abled, you will find the extra height provided by a raised bed helpful. In addition, raised beds allow you to vary the soil mixes and fertilizers used for different plants, and you can even add rodent netting under raised beds to block tunneling animals.

A framed raised bed keeps the soil from eroding and creates a tidy area for growing. Many growers make wood frames from 2 x 4s, wooden boards, concrete blocks, or recycled materials such as bricks, broken up concrete, and rocks. After you have set your framing, line the bottom with a few inches of gravel for drainage, if needed, and fill the bed to within several inches of the top of the frame using soil you've collected, a purchased planter's mix, or a mix of compost and soil. Raised beds are easiest to care for when their maximum width is between 4 and 5 feet, so that you can comfortably reach the middle of the bed without having to stand or walk on the soil.

Vertical Gardening

If your outdoor space is limited, grow up! There are many ways to grow vertically, from living wall installations to free-standing columns, arbors, suspensions, and trellises. Vines, such as honeysuckle and hops, are ideal for vertical gardening. Living walls allow you to set nonvining, clumping plants along the length of your support, resulting in a lovely cascading effect.

Cold Frames

A cold frame is like a minigreenhouse that can be used to protect tender plants from the biting cold or a possible frost, or can protect seedlings in the early spring. Portable cold frames are generally low, bottomless boxes, with sides made of wood and a glass or plastic top that allows light to enter and warmth to collect inside. (They are available online in kit form or even fully assembled.) You can further insulate the sides with hay bales or other thick materials when temperatures drop. The back of the cold frame should be 4 to 6 inches higher than the front, so the lid slopes forward and maximizes the amount of light that reaches the plants inside. Face the cold frame toward the south for the greatest sun exposure and thus the greatest amounts of heat and light. It can be moved around your garden and can be as large or small as you find useful. As the weather warms, you can prop open the lid, swing it open fully, and eventually remove the frame. A cold frame can often add a month or more to each end of the growing season, and in warmer climates it can enable gardeners to grow plants outdoors throughout the winter.

The Potted Garden, Indoors or Out

If you have a rooftop corner, a sunny breakfast room, a warm sunporch, an attached greenhouse or atrium, a deck, a porch, or a kitchen windowsill, you can grow herbs successfully. There are a number of medicinal herbs that do remarkably well in pots and planters. In fact, growing this way can allow you to cultivate botanicals that you couldn't otherwise grow in your climate and can dramatically extend your season.

Choose Your Space

Naturally, your type of residence may determine the type of potted garden you can create. But don't limit yourself; think creatively when designing spaces to incorporate herb growing into your daily care routine.

Windowsills

As long as you have enough sun streaming in through your window or can provide artificial light suspended directly

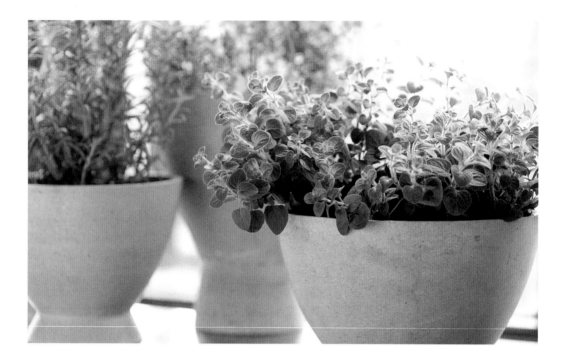

over your plants (for when the sun's angle is low, in winter, or if the window is on a northern wall), you can successfully grow herbs. You'll have to pay attention to the sun pattern, noticing when the light is direct and indirect. More than 2 to 3 hours of direct sunlight on the herbs daily will mean that you'll need to water and feed the plants more often. Without enough light, however, your herbs will become leggy and their growth will be soft and lax. Believe it or not, the biggest mistake people make with windowsill growing is neglect.

In a very sunny window, you can experiment with setting pots of herbs in a tray filled with stones and adding water to the tray. (The stones prevent the water from soaking directly into the pots, so take care that the water level doesn't reach the pots themselves.) This technique provides some humidity, which cuts down on the dramatic effects of direct sunlight. Check your pots morning and evening, and let them dry out before watering, but don't allow the plants to wilt. See page 119 for soil mixes and fertilizers you can use.

Decks and Porches

Lucky you—you have the closest thing to a land-based garden and can style it any way you wish with containers. (We provide guidelines for selecting pots on page 118.) You might want to place a potting bench in one corner of the space, so you have somewhere to work on your plants.

Decks and porches have sun and shade patterns that can be stark and change rapidly, which can create a challenge for plants until they adjust to the new space. Reflections from walls, glass, and water features can add to the effect of sun and shade, so spend some time closely observing the changing patterns to determine where on your deck or porch the shade-loving herbs should go and where to place the sun lovers.

If you work outside the home or are gone for long periods of time, you'll have to pay special attention to your plants' watering requirements. Some people set up drip irrigation tubes with timers to allow for consistent moisture and lessen plant maintenance time.

Greenhouses, Atriums, Sun Porches, and Four-Season Rooms

These indoor growing areas are full-service rooms, where you can grow in containers or make use of beds, benches, tables, or boxes. Having a true greenhouse is a luxury. If you are blessed with enough space to construct a greenhouse (or can purchase a ready-to-assemble kit online), you'll have flexibility and variety in your gardening activities. You'll be able to start seed in very early spring, long before you would be able to plant outside, and you'll be able to house tender perennials over the winter months. Greenhouses do have ongoing costs—such as heating, ventilation, and lighting—that should be factored into your buying decision. But if you live in a warm climate, you may be able to make use of an unheated greenhouse. For enthusiastic gardeners, greenhouses are indispensable, but the costs of building and maintaining one can be considerable. If you're considering a greenhouse, you could start with a temporary or "pop-up" model; they're available as lightweight kits that snap together, and they can be assembled and disassembled easily.

A more practical approach to indoor growing may be an atrium, or attached greenhouse, built onto an outside wall of your home. It will allow you to heat and light the growing area separately from the rest of the house, and it will bring in extra solar heat in the winter as an added benefit. It's ideally positioned on the south wall, and it may be less expensive to build and maintain than a traditional greenhouse. You can even purchase various designs as kits. Work with a qualified expert to help you weigh size, floor plan, lighting (such as fluorescent, LED, high-intensity discharge, or a combination), and air-quality considerations.

The next best indoor option is a roomy sunporch or glass-walled room, as long as you can provide supplemental heat and light when needed. Light is the only limitation to indoor growing; without enough light, your herbs will become leggy and start to topple. The most ideal setting will be a south-, east-, or west-facing window, although you need to factor in shade from outdoor trees and neighboring buildings.

Rooftop Growing

If you're living in a high-rise, you'll find an enthusiastic club to join—a whole set of rooftop gardeners enjoying the benefits of vegetables and herbs in planter boxes, wine barrels, old bathtubs, and even plastic kiddie pools. The possibilities are endless. Before attempting a rooftop garden, you'll need to research any local restrictions your building or town may have in place, and you should check with an expert who can advise you about structural issues that may arise from the extra weight you'll be adding to the roof. We know of buildings that have needed to be reinforced, so proceed cautiously. Once those steps have been taken, you'll need to make decisions about water sources, bed and container design and placement, and drainage, as well as determine how to deal with weather extremes your plants may face (such as high winds or intense heat) and how to bring your supplies to the rooftop.

Selecting Containers

Decorative pots, barrels, and tubs are beautiful and convenient, and there are multitudes of styles. They lend instant color and provide a focal point for the space, whether indoors or out. The only tricky thing is getting a sense of how large a pot you'll need for a particular herb, so check each herb's profile to determine its mature size. For outdoor growing, keep in mind that it's easier to grow plants in large containers than small ones because large containers hold more soil, which stays moist longer and is less subject to temperature fluctuations. For most herbs, the ideal container provides enough room for the herb to grow in one season. (For example, place an herb purchased in a 4-inch pot into a 6- to 8-inch pot.) Check the herb's profile to see how big it's going to get during the season, and use that as your guide.

You should also consider the size and shape of a plant's root system, how rapidly it grows, and whether it is a perennial, annual, or shrub. It is especially important to check your pots occasionally to make sure the root systems haven't outgrown their lodgings. Rootbound plants, which have filled up every square inch of the soil available, dry out rapidly and don't grow well.

Of course, the sizes of the containers you use will be limited by the space you have available (especially indoors), what structures or furniture will support the containers, and whether the containers will need to be moved.

Whichever container you choose, drainage holes are essential. Without drainage, soil can become waterlogged and plants will suffer. With the exception of ceramic-type pots, you can always drill drainage holes yourself. There are also self-watering, double-walled containers and pots on the market, and these are ideal for smaller plants that need frequent watering.

When choosing pots for herbs, you also need to take into account the differences between plastic, clay (such as terra-cotta), glazed ceramic, and wooden pots. Plastic warms up fast (not an advantage outdoors in areas where summers are hot and dry) and thus dries out quickly, but it's lightweight and inexpensive. Terra-cotta containers can be attractive and inexpensive; they do transpire moisture through their walls, but they also dry more evenly than plastic. You'll need to protect terra-cotta pots in colder climates because they can crack or break as they freeze and thaw. Glazed ceramic will retain moisture but can keep plants soaked with water if the drainage holes are not adequate. Wood is natural looking in an outdoor setting and can protect roots from rapid temperature extremes. Polyurethane foam pots are gaining in popularity because they resemble terra-cotta pots but are considerably lighter. However, we do not recommend growing your medicinal plants in this type of material because the toxic hydrocarbons emitted by the foam can enter your herb's roots. There's one thing to remember, no matter which type of pot you choose: Start with small pots when the plants are young and small, allowing for at least one season of growth.

Let's Plant Herbs

Once you've made decisions about the placement and possibilities of your setting, you're ready to select soil mixes and plants. Maybe you already know which herbs you'd like to grow or you're inspired to try a new plant, based on the herbs featured in this book. Consult "Plants to Grow for Herbal Healing" on page 136 to choose plants based on their preferences for shady or sunny spots, suitability for indoor growing, or soil and water preferences. After you've ordered your seeds or plants, you can get started and enjoy the beauty of medicinal herb growing.

Soil Mixes for Containers

A soil mix needs to do two things: hold the plant's roots in place and retain the nutrients and moisture it needs. As you learn about the herbs you'd like to grow, you'll notice that they have differing nutrient and moisture needs. Herbs that originate in four-season climates and the tropics will appreciate rich soil mixes, and desert or Mediterranean plants will respond better to lean soil mixes.

You can create your own soil mix with just a few garden components. Start with a base of whichever you have on hand, either good topsoil or purchased potting soil. Mix the ingredients in a large tub or wheelbarrow, or on a tarp, and then transfer it to your containers.

☀ Rich Soil Mix

You can purchase all of these ingredients (except the garden soil) at garden or farm supply stores. Coir (shredded coconut hulls) is a great substitute for nonrenewable peat, but coir dries out very quickly, so make sure it is moistened before adding it to your mix.

> 2 parts garden soil or purchased organic potting soil
>
> 2 parts compost
>
> 2 parts coir, composted fine bark, perlite, or moistened vermiculite*
>
> 1 part horticultural sand
>
> Optional: 1 to 2 parts aged manure, for outdoor mixes

*Reduce by half if you're using potting soil.

☀ Lean Soil Mix

> 2 parts garden soil or purchased organic potting soil
>
> 2 parts sand, perlite, or vermiculite
>
> Optional: 1 to 2 parts coir or other tilth-building ingredient, such as coffee grounds or peanut or rice hulls

A variety of "soilless" mixes are available. They often contain peat, which is an endangered, nonrenewable resource (although it's a superior component of soil mixes). Check before purchasing soilless mixes, and always buy a certified organic mix unless you trust the source.

You can also make your own soilless mixes.

☀ Rich Soilless Mix

> 2 parts coir, moistened
>
> 2 parts compost
>
> 1 part sand
>
> 1 part aged manure or a combination of blood meal, fish meal, bonemeal, or seaweed meal
>
> Optional: 1 part perlite or vermiculite

✳ Lean Soilless Mix

4 parts coir, moistened

2 parts sand

Optional: 1 part perlite or vermiculite

Moisten with fish emulsion, algae, or seaweed liquid (such as Maxicrop).

Potting Up Herbs

If you've purchased plants, fill your empty container half full of your soil mix and gently lift a plant out of its nursery pot by cradling the base of the plant stem between two fingers, turning the pot upside down or sideways, then tapping, squeezing, and easing out the plant. Set it in place in the container. Fill the pot with soil mix, making sure that the soil level is at least an inch or two below the rim of the container and the soil is even with, or slightly higher than, the original soil level of the plant. Firm the soil around the plant.

If you're starting herbs from seed, fill seedling trays, nursery or paper pots, or clean, recycled containers with seed-starting mix, and directly sow seeds into the mix, following the directions in the individual herb profiles. Read "Starting Seeds" on page 122 for more information.

Caring for Container Plants

Once you've invested time in planting containers, you'll want the herbs to grow well and look their best. Follow these tips for great results.

- Don't place a layer of gravel or broken pottery at the bottom of your container, as many sources recommend. That practice actually worsens bad drainage, instead of improving it.

- Water container plants thoroughly, but don't overwater! It is sometimes tricky to determine whether more is needed, but you should keep in mind that most herbs in containers should nearly dry out between waterings. You can't always tell by feeling the soil surface whether the soil throughout the container is dry, but you will want to let the plant get (almost!) to the point of wilting before you douse it.

- Container plants need regular feeding. If the herb likes rich soil, water it with a liquid fertilizer every week or two, just until the fertilizer begins to drain out of the bottom (see "Nutrients" on page 110). If it thrives in poorer soil, feed it once a month.

- Remove dead leaves and spent blossoms, and prune back plants that get leggy or stop blooming. Don't be afraid to dig out or remove plants that don't grow well or that succumb to diseases or pests.

- If the roots of a plant start to emerge from the drainage holes at the bottom of its container, it's time to repot! Use a pot that is the next size up, fill it halfway with your soil mix, place your plant in the pot, and continue filling until the soil level is a little bit higher than the original soil level of the herb. Firm the soil around the plant. Sprinkle a little bit of compost on the soil surface, then drench it with a diluted fish emulsion, seaweed, or algae fertilizer; you can also apply compost or comfrey tea.

- Plan to repot your perennial herbs every year. Each spring, remove the entire plant and its soil from the pot, and shake off any soil that comes away easily. If no soil comes off easily (or if you see the plant's roots coiled tightly around the edge of the rootball), it's time for a bigger pot. Trim away any old, dead plant material and gently loosen any visibly coiled roots. Put some new soil in the bottom of the pot (or, if you're transplanting into a larger pot, half fill the new container), set the plant on the soil, and add more soil around the sides of the plant. Then water the new transplant with liquid fertilizer.

- If your plant is too big to repot, tend and feed it yearly. Using a trowel, break up the surface of the soil and water it with comfrey tea, compost tea, fish emulsion, or other liquid fertilizer. Then apply a fresh layer of compost—as much as possible, while making sure that your soil level remains at least an inch or so below the rim of the container.

- In autumn, cut back perennial herbs and reduce your watering schedule.

Remove the top layer of compost from your pots and replace it. Bring your tender plants inside before the first frost date. You can leave hardy perennials outside, but group them together against a sheltered wall and mulch them. If severe weather is predicted, cover the entire group of pots with a thick layer of straw or leaves, string with non-LED Christmas lights, or use blankets or other protection.

- Hanging baskets make great herb containers, but be sure to place them in an easy-to-reach spot so they don't suffer from neglect. They're best located where they won't get full sun all day and won't experience high winds. Creeping herbs, such as gotu kola and oregano, are the best choices for hanging baskets. Check them every morning and evening to see if they need water.

Buying and Ordering Plants

If you're not able to start plants from seed, or you're new to gardening, purchasing plants is the way to go. You'll find a great selection of the most common herbs at your local garden center, and all of the herbs featured in this book are available at garden centers, through mail-order nurseries, or online.

Buying plants in your locale is easy, convenient, and foolproof. Because you have a chance to inspect the plants before you purchase them, you can choose healthy plants that show signs of new growth, are pest- and disease-free, and aren't rootbound. Start with just one or two plants of your selected herb to see how well they do in your conditions; you can always shop for additional plants later in the season or the following year.

If you decide to order plants from online sources, read the nurseries' advice for receiving and planting your herbs *before* you place your order. Most plants must be planted quickly after they arrive, so you'll need to be sure that you've prepared your garden or containers in advance.

Propagation

Seeding is our favorite form of propagation. A seed is a repository for all the genetic diversity of the ancient wildness of these potent medicinals. When you are looking for medicine in an herb, you want to use the purest, strongest strain of the species you can get; in other words, you want the original, unchanged, wildest form available. So you will not, in most cases, choose a hybrid, which is indicated by a multiplication sign between a plant's genus and species names or by a proper name within single quotes, like 'Jenny'. And you won't choose varieties developed for a wide array of flower colors or disease resistance. Seeds of unselected, wilder species will give you the full range of biodiversity possible for the herb— which makes it perfect for use as herbal medicine.

Most of the herbs featured in this book can be easily sown from seed. You'll find instructions for the other propagation methods (stem cuttings, root cuttings, root division, and layering) starting on page 125.

Our favorite seed sources are listed in Resources (see page 218). We recommend that you seek out certified organic sources or get to know the seed company's practices personally. We support small, local seed exchanges and regional seed houses whose activities are transparent, and we avoid those that trade in genetically modified or engineered seeds or plants.

Starting Seeds

There are a few herbs that germinate best when they are seeded directly in the garden (see the individual herb profiles in the Know It chapter). However, most get a better start when sown indoors or in a greenhouse. You can start seeds in purchased seed trays or flats, recycled plastic nursery pots, or just about anything you have available that's an appropriate size and shape: egg cartons, half clamshells, or paper cups, for example. If you can, start seeds in containers with individual cells. That way, when it's time to transplant, you won't have to disturb the seedlings' roots as much as you would while separating seedlings started in a large container.

Seed-Starting Mix Recipes

You can purchase an organic seed-starting mix at most hardware or garden stores, or you can make your own. Here are a few sample recipes.

❋Seed-Starting Mix I

1 part organic potting soil

1 part perlite or vermiculite

❋Seed-Starting Mix II

1 part garden soil

1 part well-sifted organic compost

2 parts horticultural sand or a combination of sand, perlite, vermiculite, and coir

❋Seed-Starting Mix III

1 part well-sifted organic compost

1 part perlite or vermiculite

1 part coir

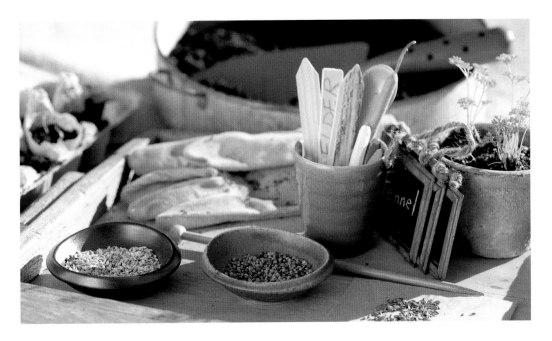

How to Plant Seeds

Follow these instructions for sowing and nurturing your newly planted seeds.

1. Make sure your mixture is moist but not soggy. Fill your clean, disinfected containers with the mix, and lightly tamp it down to settle and firm it.

2. Make a shallow indentation with your finger or a pencil or chopstick and drop in several seeds. Unless you're planning a huge garden, don't sow all of the seeds in a packet; save some for a second sowing or the next season. In most cases, the average individual or family will only need 5 to 20 plants of a particular herb.

3. Cover the seeds lightly with the seed-starting mix to a depth of two to three times the diameter of the seed. Very small seeds will get just the barest cover or will be pressed into the soil surface.

4. Water or mist the flat or container gently, label it with the name of the herb and the date, and place it in a warm location. If you are starting seeds early in the spring and the seeds need warm soil to germinate, you may want to purchase heating cables or pads (available online), or place the containers near a radiator or heater. A bright east- or west-facing windowsill with indirect light can suffice for germination. Most seeds germinate best between 60° and 80°F.

5. Label each herb container or tray with the herb name and the date. Keep the seedlings gently watered or misted so they remain moist but not soggy. (And if you'll be gone for the better part of each day, cover the containers or trays with sheets of plastic wrap or plastic bags to keep in warmth and moisture. Once the seeds have germinated, remove the covering.) Make sure new

Propagation Terminology Explained

Seed-starting is one of the easiest and most enjoyable parts of gardening, but some seeds require special consideration and procedures to ensure germination.

Cotyledon: The first leaf or one of the first pair of leaves to unfold as a seed germinates. Cotyledons generally do not resemble the plant's actual leaves.

Damping off: A fungal disease that causes seedling stems to shrivel and collapse at the soil level.

Dark-dependent germinators: Seeds that need a light barrier in order to germinate. Most times, if there's not quite enough darkness, the germination level may be reduced, but many seeds will still germinate.

Germination: The initial growth of a seed.

Inoculant: A bacterial microbe, usually found in powder or liquid form, that is applied directly to seeds in the Fabaceae (legume) family to improve germination.

Light-dependent germinators: Seeds that require light to germinate. These seeds are pressed onto the surface of the soil and kept moist until germination occurs.

Multi-cycle germinators: Seeds that require a warm cycle, a cold cycle, and another warm cycle before they will germinate. This can sometimes require more than a year for germination.

Rooting hormone: A synthetic version of a natural plant hormone that can encourage root formation on stem cuttings. Commercial rooting hormones are available in garden

---

emerging seedlings get 6 hours of sunlight daily. If they don't, you'll need to supplement with fluorescent, LED, or grow lights. Germination times vary from several days to several weeks.

6. The first leaves that emerge with germination (called the cotyledons) will be followed by the "true leaves," which will look more like the mature leaves of the herb. You can transplant a plant to its own container or an outdoor bed after the true leaves have appeared,

but it's best to wait until there are several sets of true leaves and the plant looks healthy and strong.

Transplanting Outdoors

If you're starting seeds indoors, sow them 4 to 6 weeks before the last spring frost date in your area. Once the frost date has passed, you can safely transplant seedlings into outdoor pots or beds.

As you notice that the young plants are ready, take them outdoors in their seed-starting trays or containers for a few centers and online in powder form, but they are not approved for organic use. (See "Stem Cuttings" below for an alternative.)

Scarification: The process of abrading the seed surface to make it more permeable. Some seeds have hard seed coats that need to be broken down so that they can germinate. In nature, this happens when they pass through the digestive tract of an animal or are exposed to rough, changeable weather conditions. You can mimic this process by gently rubbing the seeds with sandpaper, nicking them with a sharp knife (if they're large enough), or dropping them in boiling water and then letting them cool to room temperature.

Seed: A plant embryo and its supply of nutrients, often surrounded by a protective seed coat.

Seedling: A young plant grown from a seed.

Stratification: Exposing seeds to a period of cold to break dormancy. Cold stratification helps germinate seeds that would naturally go through freezing temperatures in the winter. You can either sow in the fall and leave the flat outdoors, where it will experience the natural rise and fall of the seasonal temperatures, or, if your winter is not frigid, you can artificially create those cool conditions: In a plastic bag, mix the seed with moist sand or vermiculite, label the bag, and place it in the refrigerator for at least 3 to 4 weeks. You can also place the bag in the freezer occasionally to simulate winter weather.

days, and bring them back inside before nightfall. This process is called "hardening off," and it helps the plants get used to the temperatures and conditions outside. After several days of hardening off, leave the plants outside overnight. Then transplant them into beds or containers, preferably in the late afternoon or on a cool day. If they're going into the ground, dig a hole bigger than the seedling and place a handful of compost or aged manure at the bottom. Place the seedling into the depression and firm the soil around it, burying the main stem slightly deeper than it had been growing in the seed-starting medium. Water it gently.

Stem Cuttings

If you have access to a mature plant of the species you'd like to grow, in many cases you can propagate by stem cuttings. Cuttings will result in a new plant in a matter of weeks, and you'll have a success rate of 50 to 90 percent, depending on the herb. Cuttings are best taken in spring or early summer.

Here's how.

1. Make a mixture of 1 part sand and 1 part perlite, or 1 part sand and 1 part moistened coir, with an optional smattering of compost tossed into the mix, and moisten it until it is wet but not soggy. This will be your rooting medium.

2. Fill clean, sterilized pots with the mixture, leaving an inch or so at the rim of the pot. Use your little finger, a pencil, or a chopstick to poke a 2-inch-deep hole in the mix for each cutting you will be starting.

3. Snip a 4- to 6-inch section of a healthy stem, and remove all leaves from the bottom one-third to one-half of the cutting, leaving only naked stem on that portion. You may also pinch off the tiny tip of the cutting.

4. As an option, you can dip the lower half of the stem cutting into rooting hormone or a strong tea made from willow bark or twigs. Insert the cutting into the hole you've poked in the rooting medium. Make sure the area you stripped of leaves is below the soil.

5. Check the moisture level of the rooting medium once or twice daily. You can also place a plastic bag over the stem cutting, making sure it doesn't touch the leaves. (Insert a bent coat hanger, chopsticks, or another support around and above the cutting.) Then cut slits in the bag to allow fresh air to reach the plant.

6. Place the cutting in bright but indirect light. If the air temperature is going to fall below 65°F, consider adding bottom heat (in the form of heating coils or pads) for greater success.

7. Stem cuttings will form roots in 2 to 4 weeks. After 2 weeks, check to see if the cutting has rooted by gently tugging on its top leaves to see if there is resistance, which is a sign that roots have formed!

8. As soon as possible after you verify that the cutting has rooted, transplant the seedling into a pot or its permanent location in the ground.

In the fall, you can take hardwood cuttings from woody plants during their dormant period. Mid-autumn is often the best time to collect and plant cuttings, because the plants will have time to form roots before buds begin to grow.

1. Make a mixture of 1 part sand and 1 part perlite, or 1 part sand and 1 part moistened coir, with an optional smattering of compost tossed into the mix, and moisten it until it is wet but not soggy. This will be your rooting medium.

2. Fill clean, sterilized pots with the mixture, leaving an inch or so at the rim of the pot.

3. Collect 4- to 8-inch cuttings from vigorous, 1-year-old wood, a few inches below the tip of the branch or stem. Make a sloping cut at each tip, slightly above a bud, and a straight cut at each base, slightly below a bud.

4. Place the cuttings 2 to 4 inches apart in the medium, with the top bud of each about 1 inch above the rooting

medium's surface. Be sure the cuttings point upward, and double-check that you've stuck the ends with straight cuts into the medium.

5. Place the cuttings (along with their rooting medium mixture) in a "nursery" trench that you've dug in the ground soon after you harvest them from the mother plant. This trench will allow them to overwinter before they're planted individually in the ground. Cover the cuttings with 6 to 8 inches of mulch.

6. Keep the cuttings moist over the winter. Remove the mulch and move your rooted cuttings to their new homes in the spring.

Root Cuttings

Plants that have taproots (like carrots) are best divided by actually taking slices from the root of the mature plant. This method also works well for plants that have long, creeping roots, rhizomes (underground stems with a rootlike appearance), or runners.

1. Dig the root carefully and gently brush off any excess soil.

2. If the plant has a taproot, cut off 1-inch slices. If you have a thin creeping rhizome, notice the growing nodes (bumps or lines on the root) and divide the rhizome into sections that each have at least two of these nodes.

3. Using the same potting mix that you would for stem cuttings, fill a pot one-half to two-thirds full. Lay the taproot

Dealing with Pests and Diseases

Herbs are generally less troubled by pests and diseases than many other garden plants are, but they can still develop problems. Vigilance is key—if you see a problem, take action right away.

You can hand-pick and remove pests, if they're big enough. Some insects, such as aphids, can be controlled with a strong stream of water. In some cases, you can apply floating row covers to discourage pests. And there are commercially available organic sprays and controls at your local garden center that will control various pests and diseases. Consult your Cooperative Extension Service about beneficial insects in your region and the herbs (such as dill and fennel) that attract them.

If you spot a disease on an annual herb, the best course of action is to remove the infected plant before the disease spreads. For perennial herbs, you can prune stems and branches at the first sign of disease. If you need further intervention, check online to find safe and organic solutions.

or thin root section on the surface and cover it with more potting mix, to just below the rim of the pot. Don't compress the soil.

4. Label your new starts and water them well.

5. When you notice a new plant emerging from the soil surface, you can transplant it into its permanent home.

Root Division

Sometimes the best way to gain a new plant is to take advantage of someone else's excess! There are quite a few plants that expand and spread by runners (underground stems) and others that self-seed profusely and form massive plantings. These can be lifted out of the soil and divided, and the resulting sections can be replanted. The same process can renew an older plant that has died out in the center. It's done with perennial herbs that have fibrous roots (as distinguished from taproots) anytime during the growing season, but is perhaps best done in the fall, when the plants are beginning to die back, or in the early spring, when growth is starting to explode. Of course, check the individual herb profiles to make sure that the herb you are working with is suited to this technique.

1. Carefully dig and lift up the whole plant, making sure to get as much of the rootball as you possibly can. If the plant is large or unwieldy, you may want to prune it to a manageable size first.

2. Shake off any excess soil and gently tease the root mass apart, sensing where it most easily wants to separate.

3. If the root is large, hard to separate, or very dense, you can use a weeding tool, a digging fork, or even clippers or scissors to separate the roots.

4. Replant all sections immediately, either into pots or in the garden. If the herb likes a richer soil, fill the new holes with compost to give the divisions some nutrition for the journey to maturity.

5. If you haven't already, prune the aboveground portions by at least half, so that the newly disturbed roots won't have to feed as much plant matter.

6. Water thoroughly.

You can also use this same technique to separate offsets and side shoots from parent plants. Remove younger, smaller shoots from the outer edges of a rootball by breaking or cutting them off, making sure that each piece you remove has its own root system. Replant the offshoot immediately to the same depth as the original plant, and water it thoroughly.

Layering

This is the oldest method of propagation, and it's one that happens naturally as certain herbs age. The long, leggy stems of some plants droop down and rest on the soil, and where they touch at a node (a raised area on the stem where the leaf attaches), roots will form. You can mimic this process by layering selected plants to create offspring.

1. Choose a strong, healthy stem, and notice where it will easily dip to the earth. Remove all the side shoots and leaves from a 6- to 12-inch section at the point of soil contact.

2. If you wish, you may use a knife to gently scrape the underside and outer woody portion of the stem for 1 to 2 inches at the point of soil contact.

3. Fluff or rough up the soil where you plan to bring the stem into contact with it, mixing in a thin layer of compost or watering with liquid fertilizer.

4. Press the stem to the earth. Anchor the stem with a stake, a U-shaped piece of wire, a stone, or something similar. Mound a layer of soil over the anchored section of stem.

5. Keep the area moist. Layering is a long process, but if you start in the spring, you should be able to separate your new plant in the fall.

6. When roots form, snip off the portion that connects the new plant to the mother plant. Pot up the new plant immediately. If it's going into the ground, transplant it in the fall, or keep it in a sheltered spot and wait until the following spring.

You can use this same technique to layer potted plants, too. Pull a runner or a long stem from the mother plant, and set it on top of the soil of a new pot. Make sure it is secure, as directed above. When it roots, you've got your new potted herb already nestled in.

Harvesting

Now for the heart of the medicine! Knowing how to properly harvest your medicinal herbs will increase the potency and efficacy of the preparations you create. You'll find specific guidelines for harvesting each herb in the individual profiles, but here are some general guidelines.

Parts of Herbs

Let's understand the terminology used to describe the plant parts when harvesting.

Berries and seeds: These are the fruits of the plant, harvested when they are fully ripe (usually when they have turned a rich, deep color and have softened and matured). Rub or brush away old flower parts and the remains of calyxes (plant material between the berry and the stem), and halve larger seeds and berries to speed up their drying time.

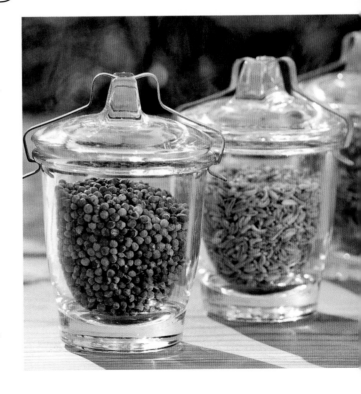

Buds: This means just the flower in its unopened state. Harvest it without any stem.

Flower: Harvest flowers by removing the whole flowering head, with little or no stem attached. The ideal time to harvest is just as the flowers are opening, but you can collect fully open flowers, as well. When they have aged to the point where their petals are drooping, however, their medicine is not as strong. Do not wash flowers unless they're visibly dirty.

Flowering tops: This term denotes the entire flowering portion of the herb, still attached to a few inches of plant stem and leaves. The tops are best for medicine when in early to full flower, and even in late flower, in a few cases (such as St. John's wort).

Herb: This refers to the aerial parts of the plant: leaves, stems, flowers, and buds (if present) and includes only the flexible portion of the stem (which usually means the top 6 to 9 inches of the plant). The herb is at its most potent when it's in early flower through the full flowering stage. Once it has started going to seed, the plant's potency has already started to decline. Don't wash herbs unless they're quite dirty. These aerial parts are usually chopped or ground for medicine making, and the thickest part of the stem is often discarded after drying.

Leaf: Take the leaf and petiole (the tender stem holding the leaf), and in some cases a very minimal amount of plant stem, if it's fleshy. Leaves that have some insect damage are fine to use, but discard those that are browning or yellowing. Dust off the leaves and lightly rinse them if they're dirty, blotting them dry before you make your medicine. Leave them whole for drying.

Root or rhizome: This refers to any below-soil roots, rhizomes (underground stems that have a rootlike appearance), and rootlet parts. You will mainly be harvesting roots of perennial, not annual, herbs. Dig them in the fall, winter, or early spring, when the plant has completely died back and all its energy has returned to the root for the winter months. If the plant is a biennial (such as angelica, burdock, and mullein), harvest from the fall after the first year of growth through the spring of the second year, before the flowering stalk shoots up. If the plant is a perennial, the best year to harvest varies with each herb; you'll find this information in each herb profile. Wash and clean roots after you dig them, cut off the crown (the point where the stem joins the roots), and either make your medicinal preparation or chop the roots into small, uniform pieces for drying.

Strobile: In the case of hops, these are the cone-shaped flowering portions of the plant. Harvest them when they're maturing from green to yellowish brown.

Whole plant: When you harvest the whole plant, you take the roots or rhizomes and rootlets (still attached to the crown), the stems, leaves, flowers, and buds—everything. The best time to harvest a whole plant is usually when the plant is in early flower. Wash the root and remove any brown or decaying aboveground portions of the plant. Then separate the aboveground and root portions for drying, since roots take much longer to fully dehydrate.

When to Harvest

Follow the guidelines above for the correct time of year to harvest each plant part. In general, the best time of day to gather any of the aboveground portions of herbs is midmorning or early evening. Start your harvest after the dew has dried but while the herbs are still cool, since excess moisture can lead to mold and blackened leaves. Herbs harvested in very hot weather or under the midday sun can bruise and wilt, causing them to lose their medicinal constituents (particularly their essential oil content). Keep them in the shade while you're collecting, and don't pile them too thickly. Roots can be harvested at any time of day that the ground can be worked, but not when there's soggy soil: You'll compact the soil and destroy all the aeration those underground critters have worked so hard to tunnel in! Remember that the soil is home to beneficial earthworms and a host of other allies.

Plan ahead: Harvest just before you make your medicinal preparations, or prepare and dry them immediately. Herbs will begin to lose potency as soon as they are harvested. Keep them in the shade while you're working, and if you need to hold them for a time, be sure to refrigerate them right away. The faster they cool, the fresher they will stay.

After harvesting, wash them as little as possible. Don't drench your herbs unless they are caked with mud or extremely dusty. You can fill a sink or bucket with water and, holding a bunch firmly, swish the tops quickly. Gently shake off the excess water and blot them dry, or lay them out on paper or cloth towels to dry.

The Right Tools for Harvesting

It's important to use the right tool for the job. Use scissors that you've dedicated to your herbs to harvest very fragile flowers,

Saving Seed for Propagation

If you'd like to save seed to start your next generation of herb plants, identify existing plants that are vigorous and disease-free. Pick their seedpods when they have dried and are beginning to fall easily from the plants, but before they become brittle or moldy.

Some plants have fragile seedpods or ripen unevenly. Loosely cover the pods of these plants with a small paper bag before the seeds have ripened completely, and twist-tie the bag snugly to the stem, so the seeds can't escape. Harvest the pods when they're fully dry, and remove the seeds. Split the pods by hand or use a wooden spoon or mallet, and collect the individual seeds.

After gathering seeds, spread them on clean paper in a warm, dry place for about a week, or place them in a roomy paper bag and shake the bag daily. Then pack them away in airtight jars and keep them in a cool, dry place.

stems, and leaves. Invest in a good-quality pair of clippers for sturdier plant parts; this will be your most frequently used tool, so buy the best. A hand trowel is versatile, especially if it has a thinner profile for maneuvering in smaller spots. If you're gardening outside, use a digging fork rather than a shovel for most root-digging harvests. A fork is gentler on the roots, lifts them out more efficiently, and disturbs the surrounding area the least.

Always use clean tools when you're digging and clipping plants. It's often recommended that clippers be dipped in a weak bleach solution and rinsed periodically to disinfect them, especially before taking stem cuttings or after pruning a diseased plant.

Drying, Preserving, and Storing

Since you can't have fresh herbs year-round, and because you don't always use everything you harvest, a drying area at home is the key to preserving your bounty and building your home medicine chest. There are three elements necessary to dry herbs effectively and safeguard their medicinal potency.

Darkness: The most crucial factor is to avoid drying your herbs in direct sunlight. Generally speaking, the darker your drying area, the better (although there are a few exceptions, such as some roots). You can use a closet, a cupboard, an old oven, an attic, or even a barn loft for drying. If you use an area in an open room, be sure to store herbs immediately after they dry, or their color (and their medicinal components) will fade before too long.

Air circulation: Choose a breezy area or keep air moving throughout the drying area so your herbs will dry evenly and quickly, before mold can grow. Even in foggy or damp weather, you can set up a fan to counteract moisture buildup. The percentage of moisture in the air should be 25 percent or less. (You can gauge it with a hydrometer.) If humidity is an ongoing problem, you may want to invest in a small, portable dehumidifier.

Heat: A steady heat source really makes a difference in the time it takes to fully dry herbs. You can set up your drying system near a woodstove or radiator or in a hot water heater closet. You can also make use of the heat rising up to your attic or into your uninsulated summer garage. Forced air dryers, such as food dehydrators, are great for small quantities of herbs, and for larger batches, you'll find plans and sample designs for electric and solar dryers online. The ideal temperature for drying most leafy plant material is 90° to 110°F; for thicker, woodier parts, the temperature can go up to 120°F. But you can dry herbs effectively at a typical range of indoor home temperatures if you have good airflow.

Drying Racks
To dry herbs quickly and evenly, set up screens or racks and lay individual leaves, flowers, berries, and root slices on them.

You'll get excellent airflow on all sides, and you can move the racks around easily. Window screens or screen doors can be set on blocks, boxes, or any kind of support. You can stretch shade cloth, netting, or fabric over wooden frames, racks, poles, or sawhorses to use as a drying surface (but don't use synthetic sheets because air doesn't pass through the fibers well). In a pinch, you can lay herbs on butcher paper or art stock spread over tables, taking care to turn and fluff the material frequently. Be sure to brush off the drying racks or other surfaces before each use to remove dust and particles from previously dried batches.

Spread your plant material thinly, without clumping or piling it. If you're planning to dry roots or other parts that need to be cleaned, wash them immediately after harvesting, pat them dry, and spread them out on your drying racks. Try to keep all of the aboveground portions of herbs as whole as possible (you can sort them after they've dried), but slice your roots to speed the drying time. Chop them into uniform-size pieces either horizontally (like carrot rounds) or vertically (like tongue depressors) if they're large enough, so they dry evenly.

Turn over the herbs daily until they're completely dry. This avoids uneven drying where plant parts overlap and pockets of moisture hide. Some very delicate flowers shouldn't be turned because they'll bruise and break, but most other leafy plants will need to be turned at least twice before they are crispy and dry.

Dehydrators

A food dehydrator is handy for drying small batches of herbs, especially leaves that are separated from their stems. It's a bit of a financial investment, but a fast and efficient food dehydrator can become the home herbalist's favorite tool.

Hanging Herbs

You can bunch long-stemmed herbs with elastics and hang them to dry. Take care not to create bunches that are too big or too dense, as this prevents air circulation in the center of the bunch, where molding can easily occur. The ideal bunch size at the elastic is the same as if you put your forefinger and thumb together in the shape of a circle. Thread a long length of twine or other sturdy line material through several bunches, like they're hanging on a clothesline, and suspend the line somewhere warm, dry, out of direct sunlight, and convenient—like your kitchen, attic, or spare room. You can suspend bunches on hooks, clothes hangers, or even on a line hung along a wall. Just be sure to store them before they fade. This method is not ideal for leafy herbs that lose their color and potency rapidly (such as spearmint, lemon balm, and oregano); be sure to store these herbs immediately after they're completely dry.

You can also place your loose herbs in paper bags and hang them in a warm or sunny place. The paper protects the herbs from light and allows air circulation. You can even punch tiny holes in the bag to increase airflow. Shake the bag every day or two so the herbs don't clump, and check them for dryness after a week. This is a great way to dry flowers and save seeds: Remove the entire flowerhead or seedhead with a nice, long stem; carefully lower it, flower pointed down, into a bag; and cinch the top of the bag loosely so debris and dust don't enter.

Oven Drying

Oven drying is a fast and slightly unpredictable method of drying herbs, yet it's a good choice if you need to dry herbs quickly or if you don't have ideal conditions to dry dense roots or big berries that might mold over time. Herbs dry very quickly in the oven, so you'll need to pay attention! Place the plant material on a cookie sheet, and turn the oven to the pilot light or lowest possible setting, taking care to leave the oven door open during the whole process. This is a touchy method, and it's easy to overdry delicate herbs because the temperature level is unpredictable.

Note: We do *not* recommend drying medicinal herbs in the microwave.

Assessing Dryness

No one who's worked hard to plant and grow herbs wants to go to the cupboard to find a gray, fuzzy mass of moldy chamomile flowers a year after putting them in storage. To avoid this scenario, you need to carefully judge the dryness of your herbs. A completely dried herb will be brittle and breakable in your hand. If stems are still bending and leaves are still pliable, they are not dry. The woody stems and denser parts of the plants will take the longest to dry, so test them first. Flowerheads (such as calendula) might seem dry on the surface, but the interior could still be damp. Press your finger all the way into the center of the flowerhead and feel for brittleness in the core of the head to be sure it's dry all the way

through. It's a common mistake to bag up calendula flowers that are not fully dry and then find the entire crop lost. Be vigilant. You'll find that atmospheric moisture will dramatically affect the final stages of drying: Herbs can reabsorb moisture overnight and be slightly damp in the morning, so wait until late afternoon to take your herbs off the drying racks so they have the heat of the day to get "crispy" dry.

Don't leave your herbs on the drying racks or hanging in bunches for too long; remove them as soon as they feel completely crispy. If they keep drying beyond that point, they'll soon brown and lose their medicinal and nutritional qualities. The end product of your efforts should resemble the living plant, both in color and texture. A good indicator of success is how recognizable your herb is as it sits in its storage container.

Fast-drying, delicate herbs generally take 3 to 5 days under ideal conditions and as long as 2 weeks in damp conditions. Roots and barks are denser and can take 2 weeks longer. Check your plants regularly, and make no assumptions about drying times.

Storing and Preserving

Once your herbs are dry, put them in storage immediately. The best storage is clean, dry, dark, and cool. Glass jars, paper bags sealed tightly shut, stainless steel (nonaluminum), and natural fiber containers work perfectly as long as they are airtight and protected from light and heat. If you need to use plastic bags temporarily, be sure the plastic is food-grade. (Avoid stiff white, gray, or black grocery bags.) Label your container with the name of the herb and the date.

Most flowers, leaves, and other above-ground portions of plants will retain their medicinal potency for a year (and in many cases, even longer) if stored correctly. Roots and barks can retain their potency for up to 2 years.

If your herbs are not carefully stored, you may find yourself with a pest problem: Mice just love dried elderberries, astragalus roots, and rose hips. Moths may get into your containers and lay eggs on drying seeds, flowers, or berries. If you find a layer of minute brown particles at the bottom of a container, with webbing or disintegrating material among the pieces, you'll have to discard your medicine. When this happens, set several insect traps in your storage area and monitor them daily. If the infestation hasn't progressed too far or you'd like to make sure a batch is protected, put the herbs in a plastic bag in the freezer for 14 to 21 days. Make sure to let the bags return to room temperature before opening them.

Keep your herb-drying and storage areas sealed off from rodents, insects, and cats looking for a comfortable place to nap. Wash your hands before handling, turning, and bagging your herbs.

Freezing is an excellent way to preserve certain herbs, if you have the space for it. They'll emerge from their frozen state somewhat discolored and mushy, but they'll smell and taste potent.

Generally speaking, this applies to leaves and fleshy roots only (such as comfrey and burdock), because flowers tend to lose their color and roots lose their texture.

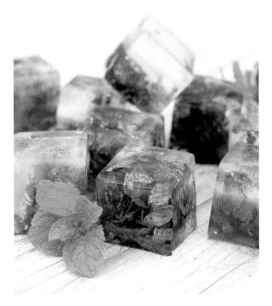

You can freeze herbs two ways. With the first method, brush off or lightly wash the leaves or roots, chop them finely, and place them in closed plastic freezer bags that are labeled with the name of the herb and the date. Use them within a year. For the second method, brush off or lightly wash the leaves or roots, chop them coarsely, pop them into a food processor or blender with enough water to barely cover them, and process them until they are finely chopped or pureed but not paste. Pour this puree into ice cube trays and freeze. When the cubes are frozen solid, break them out and put them in freezer bags. Label and date the bags, get the herb cubes back into the freezer quickly, and use them before the year is out.

Now, after months of planting, growing, harvesting, and storing, you can sit back, relax, and enjoy knowing that you've created a home medicine chest that will give back for years to come!

PLANTS TO GROW FOR HERBAL HEALING

PLANT	LIFE CYCLE	PLANT PART TO HARVEST	PROPAGATION METHOD (in order of preference)	
Aloe *Aloe vera*	Tender perennial	Leaf	Offshoots	
Andrographis *Andrographis paniculata*	Annual	Herb	Seed, cuttings, layering	
Angelica *Angelica archangelica*	Biennial	Root, seed	Seed	
Anise hyssop *Agastache foeniculum*	Tender perennial	Leaf, flowering tops	Seed, cuttings, division	
Artichoke *Cynara scolymus*	Annual or tender perennial	Leaf	Seed, offshoots	
Ashwagandha *Withania somnifera*	Tender perennial	Root	Seed, cuttings	
Astragalus *Astragalus membranaceus*	Perennial	Root	Seed	
Basil and Tulsi *Ocimum basilicum* and *O. tenuiflorum, syn. O. sanctum*	Annual	Leaf	Seed	
Burdock *Arctium lappa*	Biennial	Root, seed	Seed	
Calendula *Calendula officinalis*	Annual	Flower	Seed	
California poppy *Eschscholzia californica*	Annual	Herb, whole plant, root	Seed	
Catnip *Nepeta cataria*	Annual or short-lived perennial	Herb	Seed, cuttings, division	
Cayenne *Capsicum annuum*	Annual	Fruit	Seed	
Chamomile, German and Roman *Matricaria recutita* and *Chamaemelum nobile, syn. Anthemis nobilis*	Annual or short-lived perennial	Flower	Seed	
Comfrey *Symphytum officinale*	Perennial	Leaf, root	Seed, division	
Echinacea, purple coneflower *Echinacea purpurea, E. angustifolia*	Perennial	Leaf, flower, root	Seed	

SUITABLE FOR CONTAINER?	SOIL PREFERENCE	LIGHT/SHADE PREFERENCE	WATER NEEDS
Yes	Sandy	Sun to partial shade	Low
Yes	Sandy loam	Sun to partial shade	Moderate
Yes, though it is large	Rich loam	Partial shade to shade	Moderate to high
Yes, outdoors	Loam to sandy loam	Sun to partial shade	Moderate
No	Sandy loam	Full sun	Moderate
Yes	Sandy	Full sun	Low
No	Sandy	Full sun	Low to moderate
Yes	Average to rich loam	Full sun	Moderate
No	Average	Sun to partial shade	Moderate to high
Yes	Average	Full sun	Moderate
Yes	Average to sandy	Full sun	Low
Yes	All	Sun to partial shade	Low
Yes	Loam	Full sun	Moderate
Yes, outdoors	Sandy loam	Sun to partial shade	Moderate to high
Yes, outdoors	Average to rich loam	Sun to shade	Moderate
Yes	Average to poor	Sun to partial shade	Low to moderate

(continued)

PLANT	LIFE CYCLE	PLANT PART TO HARVEST	PROPAGATION METHOD (*in order of preference*)
Elder *Sambucus nigra, ssp. canadensis/ caerulea, syn. S. nigra, S. canadensis, S. mexicana*	Perennial	Flower, berry	Seed, cuttings, offshoots
Fennel *Foeniculum vulgare*	Tender perennial	Seed, leaf	Seed
Garlic *Allium sativum*	Perennial	Bulb	Cloves
Gotu kola *Centella asiatica, syn. Hydrocotyle asiatica*	Tender perennial	Leaf, whole plant	Layering, offshoots, division
Hawthorn *Crataegus laevigata, C. oxycantha, and C. pinnatifida*	Perennial	Leaf, flower, berry	Seed, cuttings, offshoots
Honeysuckle *Lonicera japonica*	Perennial	Flower	Seed, cuttings, layering
Hops *Humulus lupulus*	Perennial	Strobile (flower)	Cuttings, layering, division
Lavender, English *Lavandula angustifolia*	Tender perennial	Flower, bud	Cuttings, layering
Lemon balm *Melissa officinalis*	Perennial	Herb	Seed, cuttings, layering, division
Lemon verbena *Aloysia citriodora, syn. A. triphylla*	Tender perennial	Leaf	Cuttings
Licorice *Glycyrrhiza glabra, G. uralensis*	Tender perennial	Root	Seed, division
Ligustrum *Ligustrum lucidum*	Perennial	Berry	Seed, cuttings
Love-in-a-mist *Nigella damascena*	Annual	Seed	Seed
Marshmallow *Althaea officinalis*	Perennial	Root, leaf	Seed, division
Mullein *Verbascum spp.*	Biennial	Leaf, root, flower	Seed
Nettle *Urtica dioica, U. spp.*	Perennial or annual	Leaf, root, seed	Seed, division

SUITABLE FOR CONTAINER?	SOIL PREFERENCE	LIGHT/SHADE PREFERENCE	WATER NEEDS
Yes, though it is large	Rich loam to average	Sun to partial shade	Low to moderate
Yes, though it is large	Average to poor	Full sun	Low
Yes	Rich loam	Sun to partial shade	Low to moderate
Yes	Rich loam	Sun to partial shade	High
No	Average to rich loam	Sun to partial shade	Low to moderate
Yes, outdoors, if staked	Average to rich	Sun to partial shade	Low to moderate
Yes, with support	Rich loam	Full sun	Low to moderate
Yes	Sandy loam	Full sun	Low
Yes	All	Full sun to partial shade	Low to moderate
Yes	Average to rich loam	Sun to partial shade	Low to moderate
No	Average to sandy	Sun to partial shade	Low
Yes, though it is large	Average	Sun to partial shade	Low
Yes	Average to sandy	Full sun	Moderate
Yes, if the container is deep	Rich loam	Sun to shade	Moderate to high
No	Average to sandy	Full sun	Low
No	Rich loam	Partial shade to shade	Moderate to high

(continued)

PLANT	LIFE CYCLE	PLANT PART TO HARVEST	PROPAGATION METHOD *(in order of preference)*	
Oregon grape *Mahonia aquifolium*	Perennial	Root, stem	Cuttings, division, seed	
Oregano *Origanum vulgare*	Perennial	Leaf, herb	Seed, layering, division	
Peppermint and spearmint *Mentha x piperita* and *M. spicata*	Tender perennial	Leaf	Cuttings, layering, division	
Red clover *Trifolium pratense*	Short-lived perennial	Flower	Seed	
Rhodiola, Arctic rose, rose root *Rhodiola rosea*	Perennial	Root	Seed, cuttings, offshoots	
Rosemary *Rosmarinus officinalis*	Tender perennial	Leaf, herb	Cuttings, layering, division	
Sage *Salvia officinalis*	Perennial	Leaf, herb	Seed, cuttings, layering, division	
St. John's wort *Hypericum perforatum*	Annual or short-lived perennial	Flowering tops	Seed, division	
Self-heal, heal all *Prunella vulgaris*	Short-lived perennial	Herb	Seed, division	
Skullcap *Scutellaria lateriflora*	Perennial	Herb	Seed, cuttings, division	
Stevia, sweet leaf *Stevia rebaudiana*	Annual or tender perennial	Leaf	Cuttings, division, seed	
Thyme *Thymus vulgaris*	Perennial	Leaf, herb	Cuttings, seed, layering	
Turmeric *Curcuma longa*	Annual or tender perennial	Root	Division	
Valerian *Valeriana officinalis*	Perennial	Root	Seed, division	
Vitex, chaste tree, chaste berry *Vitex agnus-castus*	Perennial	Berry	Seed, cuttings	
Wormwood *Artemisia absinthium*	Perennial	Herb	Seed, cuttings, division	
Yarrow *Achillea millefolium*	Perennial	Flower, leaf	Seed, division	
Yerba mansa *Anemopsis californica*	Tender perennial	Herb, whole plant	Seed, offshoots	

SUITABLE FOR CONTAINER?	SOIL PREFERENCE	LIGHT/SHADE PREFERENCE	WATER NEEDS
Yes	Rich to average loam	Sun to partial shade	Low
Yes	Average	Full sun	Low to moderate
Yes	Rich loam to average	Sun to shade	Moderate
Yes	Rich loam to average	Full sun	Moderate
Yes	Sandy	Full sun	Low
Yes	Average to sandy	Full sun	Low
Yes	Average to sandy	Full sun	Low
Yes	Average to sandy	Full sun	Low to moderate
Yes	Average loam	Sun to partial shade	Moderate
Yes	Average loam	Sun to partial shade	Moderate to high
Yes	Rich loam	Sun to partial shade	Moderate to high
Yes	Sandy loam	Sun to partial shade	Low to moderate
Yes	Rich loam	Partial shade to shade	Moderate to high
Yes, though it is large	Rich loam	Sun to partial shade	Moderate to high
No	Average to sandy	Full sun	Low
Yes	Sandy loam	Full sun	Low
Yes, outdoors	Rich to average loam	Full sun to partial shade	Low to moderate
Yes	Rich loam	Full sun to partial shade	Moderate to high

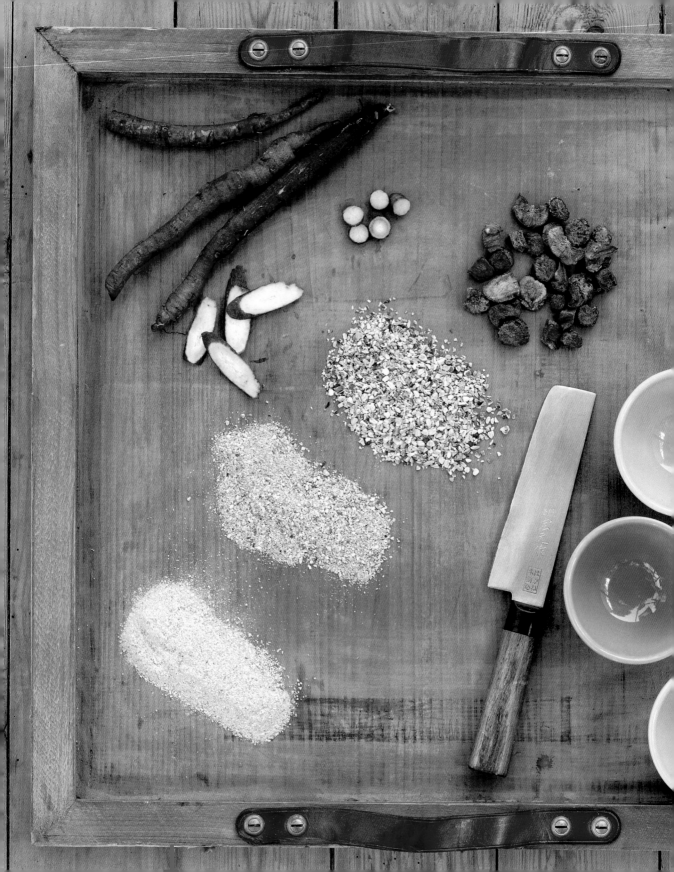

PART 3

Make It

Medicine making explained! The preparation process is rarely more complicated than mixing a recipe or making a tea. You'll choose between fresh and dried herb remedies and create many types of nature's own medicines, including tea blends, salves, creams, tinctures, oils, extracts, infusions, decoctions, compresses, and baths.

The recipes and procedures in this section are ones you'll enjoy for many years, once you discover how empowering it is to engage in self-care and why that empowerment is important to the healing process.

Perhaps you've been thinking about making your own herbal medicine, but you've had some questions. Isn't it dangerous? Don't you need lots of sophisticated equipment? And what about training? You need to be highly skilled to make your own medicines—right?

Actually, making safe and effective herbal medicines at home is an ancient tradition practiced worldwide. In many cultures, everyday ailments have been treated with handmade herbal medications for generations; in fact, only recently have medicines *not* been made in the home. Are herbal medicines safe? Yes, they are perfectly safe—especially when you prepare and use them as recommended by an experienced herbalist. The recipes and procedures in this book are ones we've enjoyed and tested for years, and the herbs suggested are time-honored and effective.

All it takes to make herbal preparations like salves, creams, and tinctures is a kitchen with common appliances like a blender, measuring spoons, and saucepans. For the more adventurous, we've included recipes for convenient dried teas, which call for a food dehydrator. If you are an experienced cook, making herbal medicines in the kitchen will feel comfortable and familiar. But even if you aren't a gourmet chef, there's no need to feel intimidated—if you can boil water, use a grater, and mix a few ingredients, you're ready. After you learn the basics of herbal preparations, you can use your imagination to create all kinds of interesting combinations.

To understand how plants heal, let's review basic plant science and the inner workings of herbs. By weight, plants are composed primarily of starches and sugars (soluble fiber), which store energy, and cellulose and lignin (insoluble fiber), which give plants their shape. Like our own bodies, plants also contain a large percentage of water. Together, these elements—the primary constituents—make up more than 95 percent of a plant.

Secondary constituents comprise the remaining 5 percent of the plant, and these are the medicinal ingredients. Even if they occur in very tiny amounts, medicinal constituents can have powerful actions. For instance, the traditional digestive herb gentian contains a compound so bitter that a single drop of the extract can be tasted in a gallon of water.

Constituents occur in different proportions in different parts of each plant. For instance, flowers are typically high in sugars like sucrose, and all aboveground plant parts contain coloring pigments like anthocyanidins and flavonoids, a plant's own "sunscreens" that protect its genetic material from ultraviolet light damage. Seeds contain unique fats to provide energy for the fast-growing sprout, and roots act as storehouses for food and medicines. Because the useful properties of plants are unevenly distributed, it's important to know where the medicinal constituents are concentrated. Another important consideration when making herbal remedies is the timing of the harvest of a particular herb, because the potency of constituents varies during a plant's life cycle. You'll find this specific information in each individual herb's profile.

What about the safety of the herbs themselves? Interestingly, when herbal treatments are compared to treatments with pharmaceutical drugs, fewer and milder side effects are usually recorded when herbal compounds are used. The preparations you'll make in these pages are some of the most time-honored and effective you can find, consistent with each herb's history of use when the plant is prepared and taken properly. Many herbs, such as ginger and garlic, are also foods that we take for their healing properties. But herbs can be harmful when misused or taken carelessly. Remember that your current physical condition and medications must be taken into consideration when choosing which herbs to take and which to avoid.

If you are experiencing or have any of the following, we recommend that you consult a qualified practitioner before preparing and using the formulas in this chapter.

- Pregnancy, anticipated pregnancy, or nursing
- A course of prescription or over-the-counter medications or other drugs
- A chronic illness
- A history of allergies
- Very young or advanced age

If you're generally in good health and are not taking life-sparing medications, such as Coumadin or chemotherapy, you'll find herbal medicines to be remarkably safe and free of side effects.

When it comes to making herbal medicines, especially teas, most people are accustomed to using dried herbs. But we hope that you'll enjoy working with the beautiful herbs that you grow and will include them in the following recipes as fresh ingredients. Fresh herbs are the most potent and desirable form of these healing plants. When an herb is dried, it loses varying amounts of its active constituents, depending on how it was dried and how long it was stored before use. But when an herb is fresh and consumed directly from the earth, it is full of "earth Qi," or healing energy. With herbs, as with food, the fresher the better.

Your Guide to Make It

In this chapter you'll find step-by-step instructions and a variety of recipes for making herbal preparations.

What You'll Need

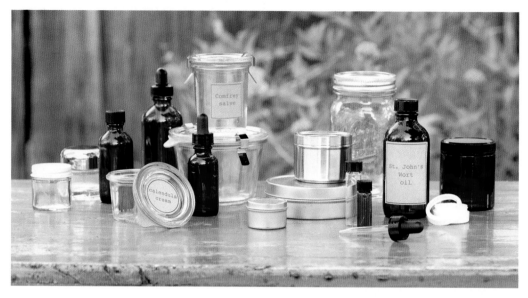

The equipment you'll need for making herbal preparations is most likely in your kitchen already. Wash all utensils, surfaces, containers, and your hands before preparing these recipes.

Pots and Pans. If you want to make effective herbal medicine, make sure you have good-quality cookware, including small and large saucepans. Uncoated stainless steel is best; don't use aluminum pans because they'll react with the active constituents, resulting in discolored or off-tasting products.

A double boiler is useful for melting wax and warming ingredients without the risk of overheating or scorching. Some people like slow cookers for melting and warming, as well as for making infused herbal oils. The gentle, steady warmth of the slow cooker (set at 100°F or "low") increases the concentration of the final oil.

Weights and Measures. Measuring cups that are made of good quality heat-resistant glass like Pyrex are excellent because the glass does not interact with the herbs. Glassware also allows you to gauge your progress by observing the color and texture of your liquid. You can judge the strength of a decoction, for instance, by how dark and rich its color is. Some ingredients, such as beeswax, are typically measured and sold by the pound or ounce, so a small kitchen scale is also handy.

Food Processor, Blender, or Grinder. Food processors can be useful for shredding fresh roots, seeds, and leafy material. Use them to chop herbs coarsely before you place them in the blender or grinder for finer grinding.

Any good blender will do the job, but if you have one with a high-speed motor, like a Vitamix, you'll be able to do a lot more with less time and energy.

The Vitamix brand has a reverse function, which helps untangle herb roots and stems from the blade, and it breaks down the plant material more thoroughly than other models. Consider purchasing a blender with a large blender jar. A 1-gallon capacity Waring blender is a good choice; it's consistently tough and efficient.

A small seed or coffee grinder is handy for grinding small quantities of dry seeds, root slices, and leaves. A good one, such as a Moulinex, often yields a finer particle size than a blender will. (Note: If you regularly need to shred whole burdock roots, dislodge seeds from really large dried flowerheads, or work with fibrous garden stalks, consider investing in a small garden compost shredder.)

Containers and Labels. For extracting herbs (removing and concentrating the active ingredient) and storing herbal preparations, you can purchase decorative jars or save and reuse glass jars from the grocery store; just be sure used jars are sterilized and have tight-fitting, rust-free lids. Canning jars are perfect: We typically use the quart or half-gallon sizes for tincturing and for storing teas and dried herbs. For creams and salves, look for smaller, short, wide-mouth containers and tins.

To bottle liquid tinctures for individual use, you'll want to purchase amber Boston rounds—those small, brown glass jars with droppers that are commonly used to package commercial herbal liquids. They come in 1- to 8-ounce sizes.

It's important to label all of your containers with the ingredients and the date. For finished preparations, be sure to include instructions for taking the herbs and any warnings that apply; put that right on the label.

Food Dehydrator. A food dehydrator is a great investment. It will dry flowers, leaves, root slices, and other herb parts quickly, while preserving their valuable constituents and colors. Of course, you can dry herbs without them (see page 132), but dehydrators can dramatically cut drying time. Many come with nylon fruit-leather tray inserts, which you'll find useful when making dried teas. If you can, buy a dehydrator with an adjustable fan speed and temperature controls.

Electric Juicer. Although a juicer is not essential for the extraction process, it increases the types of herbal preparations you can make. Juicers remove the juice from fresh herbs, which can then be used fresh or dried. You may also want to consider a hand-operated herb press, which helps squeeze out the liquid when you are making tinctures and infused oils.

Infusers and Strainers. For infusing (steeping) and straining herbs, you can simply place herbs in a tea mug, pour hot water over the herbs, and strain out the herbs after they've steeped. There are also many types of infusers and strainers, such as tea balls (mesh or metal balls that hold herbs) with handles or links that hook over the side of the mug, metal tea "spoons," bamboo tea basket strainers, muslin or mesh bags that you fill with herbs and cinch shut, and cloth bags with round rims and handles that fit on top of a mug. You can also use the same French press that many people use to brew coffee; it consists of a glass cup held by a frame with a handle and a plunger. All of these strainers make it easy to compost your herbs after you've made your tea infusion.

Teas

Tea is a time-honored and widespread preparation method used by cultures around the world today—for at least the past 3,000 to 5,000 years, as well. This makes sense, because teas utilize the most popular and available liquid substance in the world: water. Water at its boiling point (212°F) will remove, or extract, most if not all of the valuable active chemicals from an herb, concentrating them in a form that (in most cases) is safe and enjoyable to drink hot or cold. Teas are also inexpensive and cost-effective, requiring only water, a stainless steel saucepan, and a source of heat.

Here are some common questions that arise when learning how to make teas.

Is there a general herb-to-water ratio I should follow when making tea? The answer will vary, depending on how strong you want to make your tea. To make a moderately strong tea with *dried* herbs, add 1 part of a dried herb (by weight, in ounces) to 10 parts of water (by volume, in ounces); so, you'll add 1 ounce of a dried herb to 10 liquid ounces of water. You can make your tea stronger or weaker by adding more or less herb to the same amount of water—in fact, it's likely that you'll want to modify these proportions to suit your own taste. Use this 1:10 ratio as a starting point, modifying it to your liking as you continue making tea.

If you are using *fresh* herbs from your garden, add two to three times as much plant material as you would for dried herbs, meaning you'll use 2 to 3 ounces of fresh herbs to 10 liquid ounces of water.

Can I use tap water to make tea? Generally, no. When you make a tea, you should always use purified water. Tap water in some areas is fine, but other locations have water that contains unwanted chemicals such as chlorine, as well as minerals and salts that can affect the medicinal qualities of the herbs. We recommend that you have your water tested if you need to use it from the tap so you're aware of any impurities that might be present.

How long should I simmer—or boil—my tea? The answer depends on what part of the plant you are using. If you are extracting flowers, leaves, and small stems (which are thin, comparatively less dense than other plant parts, and have active chemicals that are easily and quickly extracted), you'll place them in a cup, cover them with freshly boiled water, and let them steep for 10 to 20 minutes. That's called an infusion. To strain out the herb, pour the liquid through a fine-mesh strainer and into your cup.

If you are making a tea from roots, bark, hard fruits, or seeds (which are firmer and more dense and require more time and higher heat for the active chemicals to be extracted), you'll cover the herb with water in a saucepan, bring it to a boil, reduce the heat, and gently simmer for 20 to 30 minutes (or even longer). This preparation is called a decoction. To strain out the herb, pour the liquid through a fine-mesh strainer and into your cup. Any additional tea can be stored in the fridge.

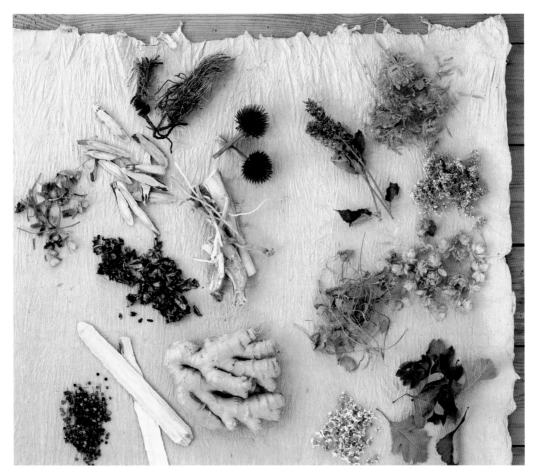

Medicinal herbs actually derive from all parts of the plant: flowers, leaves, fruits, seeds, roots, stems, and bark. Roots and bark are boiled, and flowers and leaves are steeped.

What does steeping do to herbs? Steeping herbs in water helps to release the medicinal constituents. In our opinion, hot water is the best substance for releasing the compounds stored in the cells of herbs.

What's the best way to strain herbs from tea? There is no one best way to strain herbs, but here are three options: (1) Place your loose herbs in a cup or mug, pour hot water over them, and after they steep, pour the liquid through a fine-mesh strainer. (2) Place the herbs in an infuser or strainer, and lift the infuser or strainer out of the mug when it has finished steeping. (3) Use a French press just as you would for brewing coffee, by placing your herbs in the cup of the press, pouring hot water over them, inserting the plunger to about halfway down (or well above the level of the herbs, so that you're not compressing them), and pouring the liquid out when it's finished steeping.

Can I refrigerate or store my teas for later use? Yes, you can. While we recommend that tea be consumed fresh for the best medicinal potency, you can certainly store any prepared tea in the refrigerator for up to 3 days. We prefer that you use a glass container (instead of plastic), and make sure the container is covered. See page 152 for how to make a large batch of sun tea for refrigerated storage.

Can I substitute my favorite herbs in these recipes? Certainly! Consider the recipes in each section to be starting points, and feel free to use your imagination and creativity. These are model recipes—simple templates that allow you to substitute other herbs, using the same proportions of herbs and liquid. If one doesn't seem enticing or tasty to you as you're making it, consider adding pleasant-tasting herbs such as licorice, anise, or cinnamon to the brew. Orange or grapefruit peel add flavor and are digestive aids. Stevia is a powerful herbal sweetener that helps take the edge off bitter teas, and honey combines well with most herbs. Use all of your senses to craft medicines that you love.

You'll notice that some of the specially named recipes in this chapter include herbs not covered in the 50 herb profiles. These alternate herbs are relatively common and can be found in many herb nurseries and in the bulk food departments of most natural food stores, or they can be ordered online. In some cases, we've included suggestions for substitutions. Even if you can't grow or obtain all of the ingredients, you can always use your own homegrown herbs or other herbs you have access to (and leave out any that you don't have on hand).

Infusions

Infusions are the most common way to make teas from fresh or dried leaves, flowers, or flowering tops. Use 10 liquid ounces of freshly boiled water (with the heat just turned off) for every 2 to 3 ounces of fresh herb or 1 ounce of dried herb (or, of course, a combination of fresh and dried herbs). Pour the freshly boiled water over the herb, either loose in a mug or held in a tea ball or infuser. Let it sit, covered (use a tea mug lid or "hat," a small saucer, or anything flat and nonporous so the constituents don't evaporate), for 15 to 20 minutes. Remove your tea ball or infuser or pour the liquid through a fine-mesh strainer to remove the loose herbs; compost the herbs. You can take tea in 1-cup doses at least three times daily, up to 6 cups per day, in most cases. (See the individual herb profiles for exceptions to this general rule.) For very light and fluffy herbs, like mullein or chamomile blossoms, you can increase the amount of water to make sure the herb material is completely immersed.

Gentle infusions preserve the maximum amount of volatile components, such as essential oils and other fragile plant substances. They are made by starting with room-temperature water, utilizing a smaller herb-to-water ratio, and steeping for an extended period of time. To make a gentle infusion, place 1 ounce of fresh or dried herb in a container, cover it with 4 to 10 liquid ounces of purified water, and stir to make sure the two are thoroughly combined. (For even greater extractability, you can place the herb and water in a blender or food processer and gently whir for 10 to 20 seconds on the lowest setting, and then pour the mixture into the container.) Let the mixture steep, covered, for 8 to 12 hours. Strain, using a fine-mesh strainer, and compost the herb. Drink the infusion in 1-cup doses, three to six times daily. You can experiment with the amount of water you add (between 4 and 10 parts), depending on the strength of the herb and your taste preference.

A *sun tea* is a form of gentle infusion that uses the warmth of the sun to enhance the extraction process. Place 2 to 3 parts fresh or dried herb (measured in ounces) in a clean, clear glass jar with a lid. Pour 4 to 10 parts purified room-temperature water (measured in liquid ounces) over it, and stir to make sure that the herb is completely combined with the water. Put the closed jar in a sunny place and leave it until the tea is strong enough to suit your taste (usually 4 to 6 hours). Strain the herb from the tea and enjoy the drink at room temperature or chilled. You can refrigerate sun tea for up to 3 days.

☀ Basic Infusion

There is nothing more enjoyable than gathering herbs on a warm summer morning and bringing them indoors for a refreshing cup of healing tea. Here's a sample recipe for making an infusion from the herbs that you've picked fresh from your garden or dried yourself.

> 2–3 ounces fresh or 1 ounce dried herbs
>
> 10 liquid ounces purified water

Place the herbs in a tea ball, infuser, or directly in a tea mug or other container. Bring the water to a boil. Immediately pour the water over the herbs and let the mixture steep, covered, for 15 to 20 minutes. Strain and compost the herbs. Drink the infusion in 1-cup doses at least three times daily, up to 6 cups per day.

☀ Basic Gentle Infusion

You can use this recipe with a variety of herbs, such as anise hyssop, catnip, chamomile, lavender, lemon balm, lemon verbena, oregano, peppermint, spearmint, and thyme. All of these herbs have an abundance of volatile or aromatic compounds that are ideally preserved with this method.

> 2–3 ounces fresh or 1 ounce dried herbs
>
> 10 liquid ounces purified room-temperature water

Whir the herbs and water in a blender or food processor for 15 to 20 seconds. Place the mixture in a clean, covered container and let it steep for 8 to 12 hours. Strain and compost the herbs. Drink 1 cup three to six times daily.

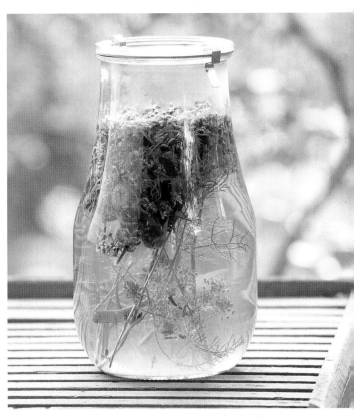

Healing herbal tea infusions can be created with the help of the sun's warmth.

✳ Basic Sun Tea

Making a sun tea is a fun and easy way to slowly infuse herbs in the sun's rays. Use this method in the summertime, when you'll have at least 4 to 6 hours of sun to warm your tea to perfection.

> 2–3 parts fresh or 1 part dried herbs, measured in ounces
>
> 4–10 parts purified room-temperature water, measured in liquid ounces

Place the herbs in a clean, clear glass jar with a lid. Add the water, and stir to thoroughly combine. Close the jar, and place it in a sunny location until the tea is strong enough to suit your taste (usually 4 to 6 hours). Strain and compost the herbs. Enjoy the drink at room temperature or chilled. You can refrigerate sun tea for up to 3 days.

Decoctions

Decoctions are made with the hard or woody parts of an herb, such as the bark, roots, and seeds. To extract all of the properties of these denser plant parts, you will need to bring the water to a boil and simmer the mixture. Start with 2 to 3 ounces fresh or 1 ounce of dried herb (or a combination of herbs), and place it in an uncovered saucepan. Add 10 liquid ounces of purified water, stir to thoroughly combine the herbs and water, and bring to a boil. Reduce the temperature and gently simmer the herbs for 20 minutes to 1 hour. Many herbalists follow the traditional Chinese decoction method, which simmers down the liquid for a longer time period, about 45 minutes to 1 hour. If you're just getting used to the bolder taste of decoctions, begin by simmering for a shorter time period, about 20 to 30 minutes or longer, increasing the time as you adjust for your taste preferences. You can take 1 cup two or three times daily.

If you'd like to make a larger amount and store it, make a quart or two of tea. For 1 quart, start with 5 cups of water and add 8 to 10 ounces fresh or 4 ounces of dried herbs. You'll lose 1 cup of water in the boiling process, and the end result will be 4 cups (1 quart). Prepare as above, bringing the mixture to a boil, reducing the heat, and simmering for your desired time period. Once again, strain the liquid and compost the herbs. You can refrigerate this for up to 3 days.

Light decoctions are appropriate for certain comparatively lighter, more porous roots, barks, and seeds (such as the stiff, thick leaves of comfrey, rosemary, and white sage; the thin roots of valerian; and the light seeds of vitex). A light decoction is prepared in a covered saucepan, which helps to prevent the escape of volatile constituents like essential oils. Begin by placing 2 to 3 ounces of fresh herbs or 1 ounce of dried herbs in a stainless steel saucepan. Pour 10 liquid ounces of purified water over them, stir to thoroughly combine the water and herbs, and bring the mixture to a boil. Reduce the heat and simmer for 10 to 20 minutes. After turning off the heat, you can let the mixture steep for another 10 to 15 minutes if you wish to further extract the active constituents, then strain and use or refrigerate the decoction. Drink 1 cup two or three times daily. Adjust the herb-to-water ratio to suit your taste.

Herbal Ice

If you want to make a large batch of medicinal tea and keep it beyond the 3-day limit in the refrigerator, let the tea cool, pour it into ice cube trays, and freeze it. Then pop out the cubes and store them in heavy plastic freezer bags, using them as needed.

Our favorite teas for freezing into cubes are echinacea (very effective against sore, inflamed throats during a cold or flu); lemon balm, lemon verbena, and lemon thyme (for digestive help and summer refreshment); and ginger and chamomile (for upset stomachs and nausea).

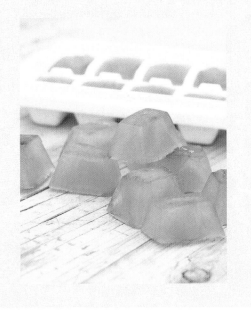

❋ Basic Decoction

Use this recipe to extract the goodness from hardy roots you've lifted out of the soil and from seeds ripened in the late summer sun. Enjoy the deep earthiness and strength of this medicinal preparation.

> **2–3 ounces fresh or 1 ounce dried root, seed, or bark**
>
> **10 liquid ounces purified water**

Grind the root, seed, or bark in a blender or food processor. Place it in a saucepan and add the water. Bring to a boil, reduce the heat, and simmer, uncovered, until the liquid is reduced by about one-third. Strain and compost the herb. Store the liquid in the refrigerator. Drink $\frac{1}{2}$ cup three or four times daily.

❋ Basic Light Decoction

Use this recipe for light roots, seeds, and barks, or for tough leaves with hard-to-extract constituents. This method is perfect for comfrey leaves, rosemary leaves, white sage leaves and twigs, valerian roots, and vitex seeds.

> **2–3 ounces fresh or 1 ounce dried plant material, as described above**
>
> **10 ounces purified water**

Place the herbs in a saucepan; pour the water over them. Stir to thoroughly combine the water and herbs, cover, and bring the mixture to a boil. Reduce the heat and simmer for 10 to 20 minutes. After turning off the heat, let the mixture steep for another 10 to 15 minutes, then strain and compost the herbs. Drink 1 cup two or three times daily, warm or cool. Adjust the herb-to-water ratio to suit your taste.

✳️Three-Seed Tummy Tea

This delicious tea is a favorite for preventing gas after meals. You'll notice that it's a light decoction followed by an infusion because of the plant parts that are included. This recipe can be made with either fresh or dried herbs; you can use a mixture, if you have some of both.

- 3 teaspoons fresh or 2 teaspoons dried cumin seed
- 3 teaspoons fresh or 2 teaspoons dried fennel seed
- 3 teaspoons fresh or 2 teaspoons dried caraway seed
- 2 teaspoons chopped fresh or 1 teaspoon dried orange peel
- 1–2 teaspoons chopped fresh or ½ teaspoon dried licorice root
- 3 cups purified water
- 1–2 teaspoons fresh or ½ teaspoon dried peppermint leaf

Place the cumin, fennel, caraway, orange, and licorice in a saucepan. Add the water and simmer, covered, for 20 minutes. Remove from the heat, add the peppermint, and let steep, covered, for 15 minutes. Strain and compost the herbs. Drink 1 cup up to three times a day. You can make a larger batch and store it in the refrigerator for up to 3 days.

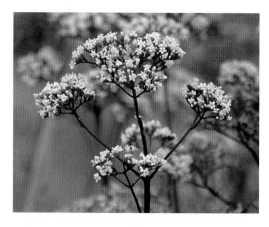

✳️Sleep Deep Tea

This is a blend of pleasant herbs to help relax your body and mind and promote a deep, refreshing sleep.

- 2–3 teaspoons fresh or 1 teaspoon dried valerian root
- 3 cups purified water
- 4–6 teaspoons fresh or 2 teaspoons dried chamomile flower
- 2–3 teaspoons fresh or 1 teaspoon dried St. John's wort flowering tops
- 2–3 teaspoons fresh or 1 teaspoon dried lemon balm herb
- 2–3 teaspoons fresh or 1 teaspoon dried hops flower
- 2–3 teaspoons fresh or 1 teaspoon dried catnip herb
- 4–6 teaspoons fresh or 2 teaspoons dried passionflower herb (optional)
- 1 teaspoon fresh or ½ teaspoon dried stevia leaf (optional, for sweetness)

Make a light decoction (see page 153) with the valerian root and water. Add the chamomile, St. John's wort, lemon balm, hops, catnip, and optional passionflower and stevia. Cover the saucepan and steep for 20 minutes. Strain and compost the herbs. Drink 1 or 2 cups before bed as desired. You can make a larger batch and store it in the refrigerator for up to 3 days.

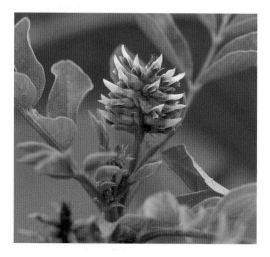

✳Cold and Flu Brew

This classic blend is comforting and healing during the misery of a cold or flu. It helps lower a fever, removes toxins from your body, fights viral infections, and acts as a decongestant. This recipe is unusual because it calls for simmering flowers to draw out special chemicals that take additional heat to extract. The recipe is formulated for fresh herbs, but if you need to substitute dried for any of them, just use half the quantity listed.

 4 teaspoons chopped echinacea leaf

 4 teaspoons elder flower

 4 teaspoons yarrow flower or leaf

 3 cups purified water

 2 teaspoons peppermint leaf

 ½ teaspoon stevia leaf
 (optional, for sweetness)

Place the echinacea, elder, and yarrow in a saucepan. Add the water and simmer, covered, for 10 to 15 minutes. Remove from the heat, add the peppermint and optional stevia, and steep the entire mixture, covered, for 10 minutes. Strain and compost the herbs. Drink up to 3 cups daily. You can make a larger batch and store it in the refrigerator for up to 3 days.

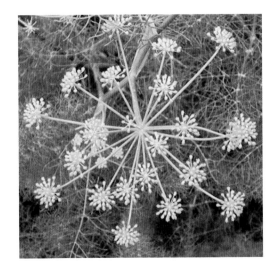

✳Cleansing Tea

This fantastic tea contains cleansing, liver-stimulating, cooling, and soothing dried herbs to reduce inflammation or irritation throughout your digestive tract, along with giving your system a good cleanse. It tastes great, too!

 4–6 teaspoons fresh or 2 teaspoons
 dried fennel seed

 2 teaspoons dried fenugreek seed
 (*Trigonella foenum-graecum*)

 2 teaspoons dried flax seed
 (*Linum usitatissimum*)

 1 heaping teaspoon grated fresh
 or ½ heaping teaspoon dried
 powdered ginger root

 ½–¾ heaping teaspoon chopped fresh or
 ¼ heaping teaspoon dried licorice root

 3 cups purified water

 ½–¾ heaping teaspoon fresh
 or ¼ teaspoon dried peppermint leaf

Place the fennel, fenugreek, flax, ginger, and licorice in a saucepan and add the water. Cover and simmer for 20 minutes. Remove from the heat, add the peppermint, and steep the entire mixture, covered, for 10 minutes. Strain and compost the herbs. Drink 1 cup three times a day or as desired. You can make a larger batch and store it in the refrigerator for up to 3 days.

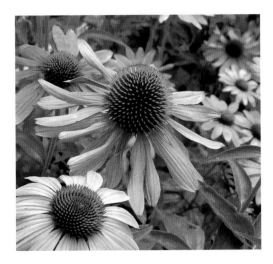

✳ Calming After-Dinner Tea

A cup or two of this relaxing and delicious infusion is the perfect ending to a satisfying meal.

2–3 tablespoons fresh or 1 tablespoon dried lavender flower

4–6 teaspoons fresh or 2 teaspoons dried lemon balm leaf

4–6 teaspoons fresh or 2 teaspoons dried chamomile flower

4–6 teaspoons fresh or 1 to 2 teaspoons dried fennel seed

2–3 teaspoons fresh or 1 teaspoon dried oatstraw or tops

1 teaspoon fresh or ½ teaspoon dried stevia leaf (optional, for sweetness)

3 cups purified water

Place the lavender, lemon balm, chamomile, fennel, oats, and optional stevia in an infuser or a container. Bring the water to a boil. Immediately pour the water over the herbs and let the mixture steep, covered, for 20 minutes. Strain and compost the herbs. Drink the infusion in 1-cup doses at least three times daily, up to 6 cups per day. You can make a larger batch and store it in the refrigerator for up to 3 days.

When Cold and Flu Season Arrives

These two recipes are prepared as teas but are not taken in your teacup—they help with the discomfort of flu season in other ways!

Winter Inhalation

This traditional herbal steam helps open your sinuses, discourages bacterial and viral growth, and reduces pain and inflammation. Remember to stay a comfortable distance from the steaming pot to avoid burning your face.

8–12 teaspoons fresh or 4 teaspoons dried eucalyptus leaf (*Eucalyptus globulus*)

2–3 tablespoons fresh or 1 tablespoon dried peppermint leaf

2–3 tablespoons fresh or 1 tablespoon dried thyme herb

3 cups purified water

Essential oils of the herbs above (optional)

Place the eucalyptus, peppermint, thyme, and water in a saucepan and stir to thoroughly combine. Bring to a boil, reduce the heat, and simmer, covered, for 5 to 10 minutes. Remove from the heat and uncover. Drape a large towel over your head and the saucepan, forming a steam-filled tent, and inhale the medicated steam deeply for 5 minutes or so. Repeat several times daily as needed, warming the decoction each time just to the boiling point.

You can enhance the inhalation by adding 6 or 7 drops of essential oil to the brew after you remove it from the heat. Try oils of eucalyptus, peppermint, and thyme, and add one or more as desired. (Because essential oils can cause dizziness and light-headedness, do not use enhanced inhalations more than two or three times a day, and discontinue use if redness of the mucous membranes develops.)

✳ Stress-Buster Tea

This infusion supports the adrenal glands and helps counteract the harmful effects of stress.

4–6 tablespoons fresh or 2 tablespoons dried chamomile flower

2–3 tablespoons fresh or 1 tablespoon dried lavender flower

4–6 tablespoons fresh or 2 tablespoons dried oatstraw or tops

6–9 tablespoons fresh or 3 tablespoons dried lemon balm herb

2 tablespoons chopped fresh or 1 tablespoon dried orange peel

1 teaspoon fresh or ½ teaspoon dried stevia leaf (optional, for sweetness)

4 cups purified water

Place the chamomile, lavender, oats, lemon balm, orange, and optional stevia in an infuser or container. Bring the water to a boil. Immediately pour the water over the herbs and let the mixture steep, covered, for 20 minutes. Strain and compost the herbs. Drink up to 5 cups a day. You can make a larger batch and store it in the refrigerator for up to 3 days.

A Soothing Throat Gargle

This decoction soothes throats that are sore from illness or hoarse from overuse; it's ideal for public speakers or teachers even when it isn't winter! You'll notice that this recipe calls for simmering aboveground portions of the plant that are usually steeped; this is because you will be extracting deeper compounds that are only somewhat water-soluble.

5–7 tablespoons fresh or 2½ tablespoons dried echinacea leaf

4–6 tablespoons fresh or 2 tablespoons dried lemon balm herb

3–5 tablespoons fresh or 1½ tablespoons dried sage leaf

3–5 teaspoons fresh or 1½ teaspoons dried licorice root

2 tablespoons dried witch hazel bark (*Hamamelis virginiana*) or marshmallow root

1½ tablespoons fresh or dried usnea lichen, if available (*Usnea* spp.)

5 cups purified water

Place the echinacea, lemon balm, sage, licorice, witch hazel or marshmallow, and optional usnea in a saucepan. Pour the water over the herbs and stir to thoroughly combine. Cover the pan, bring it to a boil, reduce the heat, and simmer for 15 minutes. Remove from the heat and steep for 10 minutes, covered. Strain and compost the herbs. You can make a larger batch and store it in the refrigerator for up to 3 days.

Gargle with ¼ cup of the warm or room-temperature tea four or five times a day; swallowing the liquid after gargling will provide extra benefits. For portability, put some in a little dropper bottle, and gargle with 3 or 4 droppersful for 30 seconds as a quick fix for an irritated throat.

✳ Immune-Support Tea

This decoction strengthens your natural immunity.

> 4–6 teaspoons fresh or 2 teaspoons dried ligustrum berry
>
> 2–3 teaspoons chopped fresh or 1 teaspoon dried astragalus root
>
> 2–3 teaspoons chopped fresh or 1 teaspoon dried shiitake mushrooms
>
> 1–2 teaspoons chopped fresh or ½ teaspoon dried licorice root
>
> 5 cups purified water

In a blender or food processor, combine the ligustrum, astragalus, shiitake, and licorice. Process the herbs coarsely and place them in a saucepan. Pour the water over the herbs and stir to thoroughly combine. Heat and simmer, uncovered, for 20 to 30 minutes. Remove from the heat. Strain and compost the herbs. Drink 1 cup three times a day as needed. You can make a larger batch and store it in the refrigerator for up to 3 days.

✳ Menopause Tea

The herbs in this light decoction have a mild estrogenic effect, regulate all the female hormones, aid in blood circulation, and have a general health-promoting effect on the female organs.

> 4–6 teaspoons fresh or 2 teaspoons dried nettle herb
>
> 2–3 teaspoons fresh or 1 teaspoon dried vitex berry
>
> 2–3 teaspoons fresh or 1 teaspoon dried ligustrum berry
>
> 2–3 teaspoons fresh or 1 teaspoon dried lavender flower
>
> 2 teaspoons fresh or 1 teaspoon dried fennel seed
>
> 2–3 teaspoons fresh or 1 teaspoon dried licorice root, or stevia herb, to taste
>
> 3 cups purified water

Optional

> 1 teaspoon dried black cohosh root (*Actaea racemosa*)
>
> 1 teaspoon dried dang gui root (*Angelica sinensis*)

Place the nettle, vitex, ligustrum, lavender, fennel, licorice or stevia, and optional black cohosh and dang gui in a saucepan. Pour the water over them and stir to thoroughly combine. Cover and bring the mixture to a boil. Reduce the heat and simmer, covered, for 15 minutes. Remove from the heat and let steep, covered, for an additional 15 minutes. Strain and compost the herbs. Drink up to 3 cups a day as needed. You can make a larger batch and store it in the refrigerator for up to 3 days.

Dried Teas

Teas (infusions and decoctions) are some of the most vital components of a self-care routine, but you aren't likely to have access to fresh herbs year-round, even if you extend your growing season by keeping some indoors in the winter. Enter the benefits of dried teas! If you're lucky enough to own a food dehydrator, you can preserve teas for future use.

First, you'll prepare a tea by decocting your favorite herbs (see page 210 to see which herbs are suitable for the dried tea process), and then you'll strain out the herbs and boil and reduce the liquid to concentrate it. Finally, you'll dry that liquid in the fruit leather trays of a dehydrator to create dried tea wafers.

Dried teas are very concentrated. Just $\frac{1}{2}$ teaspoon of a powdered dried tea contains all the active constituents of up to 5 teaspoons of the fresh herb. To use dried teas, you can eat a piece of the wafer the size of a quarter or a silver dollar, two or three times daily, or you can make an instant tea by adding $\frac{1}{2}$ to 1 teaspoon of the wafer powder to warm or hot water. These very highly concentrated extractions can be a bit strong for sensitive stomachs. If you find your blend has that effect, dilute it with more water or soothing licorice or marshmallow tea, and drink it just before mealtimes. For convenience, you can also grind your dried wafer into a fine powder and place it into 00-size gelatin capsules; the typical daily dose is two or three capsules, two or three times daily, with meals.

Follow this process to make a tea, reduce it to a concentrate and ultimately a batter, and then dry it in a food processor to create dried tea wafers. These can be thin or thick and sheet-like or flaky, depending on the herb.

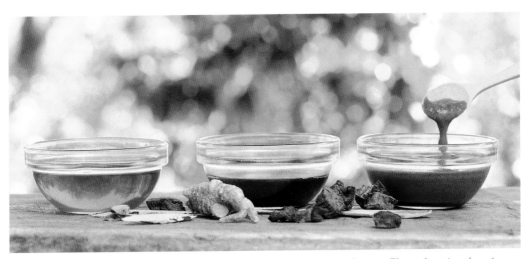

To create a long-lasting dried tea, start with fresh or dried herbs and water. Through a step-by-step steeping, simmering, and evaporating process, the tea is reduced from a clear liquid to a thick, nutrient-rich batter full of active compounds and suitable for drying.

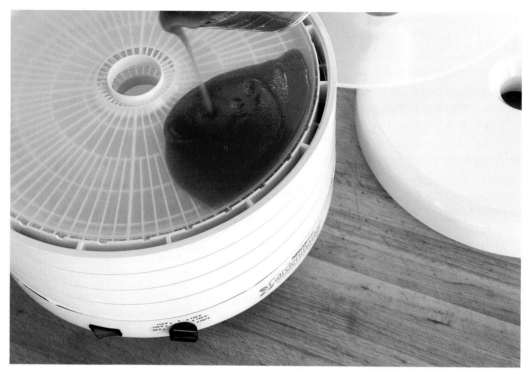

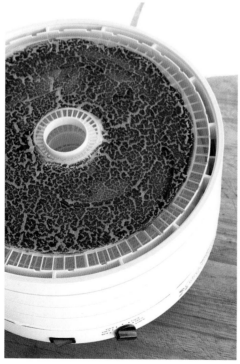

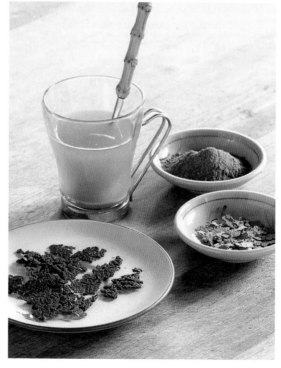

✳ Basic Dried Tea

Approximately 4 cups coarsely chopped fresh or dried herbs (more if you're using light materials like flowers and leaves and less if you're using dense materials like barks, roots, and seeds)

10 cups purified water

1–5 teaspoons "carrier," such as maltodextrin (preferred), lactose, or food-grade methylcellulose*

Place the herbs in a large saucepan and stir to thoroughly combine. Add the water and simmer, uncovered, for 2 to 4 hours or until a dark, strong tea is formed. Let it cool until it's lukewarm. Strain out the herbs and press or squeeze them as dry as possible, catching the liquid to return to the pan. Compost the spent herbs. You can strain the tea again to remove granules or sediment. Simmer the tea again until it is reduced to ½ to 1 cup of liquid. Let it cool until it's warm.**

Stir in 1 to 5 teaspoons of the carrier, until the liquid thickens to the consistency of cake batter. Pour this "batter" into the lightly oiled fruit leather trays of a food dehydrator set at 95° to 100°F. (Higher temperatures will toast the powder and reduce its quality.) Dry the liquid completely; this may take from 2 hours to overnight. When it's completely dry, the tea will be a thin, dry, solid wafer that is easily broken or powdered in a blender. Store the wafer, broken up or powdered, in an amber glass jar away from direct sunlight. Follow the dosage directions on page 159.

*You can find sources for these on page 220. You can also use a dried and finely powdered herb, such as burdock, eleuthero (*Eleutherococcus senticosus*), or nettle as a carrier. However, if you add water to your dried tea later to make a cup of liquid tea, these herbs will leave a bit of insoluble residue at the bottom of your cup.

**If you wish, tinctures of herbs such as echinacea, ginger, and orange peel can be stirred into the cooled mix before it starts to dry, either to add medicinal effects or to improve the taste. This is also a great way to add herbs such as valerian, which contains delicate essential oils and other sensitive compounds that would be destroyed by the boiling process. See page 165 for information about tinctures.

✳ Strengthen-the-Middle Dried Tea

This recipe helps strengthen your digestive system and remove excess water from your body.

¾ cup fresh or dried ginger root

¼ cup fresh or dried ginseng root, red Korean or Chinese (*Panax ginseng*)

1 cup fresh or ½ cup dried burdock root

½ cup fresh or ¼ cup dried orange peel

1 cup fresh or dried astragalus root

10 cups purified water

½ ounce tincture of artichoke leaf (optional)

Approximately ¼ cup eleuthero powder, maltodextrin, or other carrier

Place the ginger, ginseng, burdock, orange, and astragalus in a large saucepan and stir to thoroughly combine. Add the water and simmer, uncovered, for 2 to 4 hours or until a dark, strong tea is formed. Let it cool until it's lukewarm. Strain out the herbs and squeeze them, catching the liquid to return to the pan. Compost the spent herbs. Simmer the tea again until it is reduced to ½ to 1 cup of liquid. Let it cool until it's warm. Stir in the optional tincture and eleuthero powder or other carrier. Pour the batter into the lightly oiled fruit leather trays of a food dehydrator and dry at 95° to 100°F. Dry the liquid completely, and break up or powder the wafer. Store in an amber glass jar away from heat and light. Follow the dosage directions on page 159.

Bath Teas

A good warm bath at the end of a busy day—at any time, in fact—can melt away stress, treat skin irritations and muscle aches, and relieve symptoms of colds and flu. Enhance warm water's natural relaxing qualities with a strong herbal tea poured directly into the bath. Some of the medicinal constituents will be absorbed effortlessly through your skin, and others, such as volatile oils, will rise from the surface of the water with the steam and be absorbed through the mucous membranes of your respiratory tract. Keep in mind that bath teas are not formulated for internal consumption, so don't use them as beverage teas. Carefully label these teas for bathing use only, and store them near the bathroom.

Try these delightful bath tea recipes. Each one makes enough tea for a single bath and can be added either with the herbs still in the tea water or strained out.

☀ Bedtime Bath Tea

This bath tea's wonderful fragrance relaxes your spirit, and its healing substances soften your skin. It's a perfect tea for helping to calm children in the evening before bed.

> 1 heaping cup fresh or ½ cup dried chamomile flower
>
> 1 heaping cup fresh or ½ cup dried lemon balm herb
>
> ⅔ heaping cup fresh or ⅓ cup dried lavender flower
>
> 10 cups purified water
>
> Several drops essential oil such as lavender or orange (optional)

Place the chamomile, lemon balm, and lavender in a saucepan. Add the water and stir to thoroughly combine, cover, and gently simmer for 5 minutes. Turn off the heat and let it steep for 20 minutes. If desired, strain and compost the herbs or feel free to include them in your bath for extra healing benefits. Add the optional essential oil and stir well. Add the tea to a warm bath and enjoy.

☀ Healthy Skin Bath Tea

These herbs are especially soothing during gardening season, when mosquito bites, scratches and scrapes, and a little sunburn are likely.

> ½ heaping cup fresh or ¼ cup dried calendula flower
>
> ½ heaping cup fresh or ¼ cup dried plantain leaf
>
> ½ heaping cup fresh or ¼ cup dried gotu kola herb
>
> ½ heaping cup fresh or ¼ cup dried lavender flower
>
> ½ heaping cup fresh or ¼ cup dried echinacea leaf
>
> 2–3 tablespoons fresh or dried ginger root
>
> 10 cups purified water

Place the calendula, plantain, gotu kola, lavender, echinacea, and ginger in a saucepan. Add the water, stir to thoroughly combine, cover, and gently simmer for 30 minutes. If desired, strain and compost the herbs. Add the tea to a warm bath and enjoy.

Syrups

Syrups are useful for coating your throat and are helpful if you (or your kids) have trouble swallowing capsules or pills. Any herbal tea can be concentrated and added to a sweet base to create a syrup. Because this process concentrates the herb's active constituents, a syrup can be very effective at treating and healing a wide range of ailments, especially upper respiratory infections and sore throats.

After making your syrup, bottle it, label it, and store it in the refrigerator. If no preservatives are added, the syrup will probably last 2 to 3 weeks. You can add a few drops of an essential oil or vitamin C powder ($\frac{1}{2}$ to 1 level teaspoon to 1 cup of syrup) to increase its refrigerated shelf life by 1 to 2 weeks or even longer. If it's impractical to store the syrup in the refrigerator, add the vitamin C powder and grain alcohol so that the finished product is 25 percent alcohol and 75 percent syrup. These additions are particularly helpful for keeping syrup viable and safe for consumption when you're traveling. Take 1 teaspoon two to three times daily or as needed.

Sweet Syrup Bases and Herbal Syrups

Sweet Syrup Base: If you're using sugar for the sweet syrup base, you will want to make a simple syrup by dissolving 1 cup of sugar in 1 cup of water by simmering it for 30 to 40 minutes. Add this syrup to the strained tea. Add the vitamin C or alcohol and bottle, label, and store your finished syrup.

To create an alternate sweet syrup base using honey, you can combine $\frac{1}{2}$ cup each of honey and barley malt, or combine $\frac{3}{4}$ cup of honey and $\frac{1}{4}$ cup of glycerin; either of these two additions will create a smooth consistency.

Herbal Syrups: If you are including scented leaves and flowers such as anise hyssop, basil or tulsi, catnip, lavender, lemon balm, lemon verbena, oregano, peppermint, sage, spearmint, or thyme to make syrup, keep in mind that the plant material itself shouldn't be boiled. These aromatic herbs contain volatile oils that will be lost when subjected to the high heat of boiling. You will want to add them to the liquid after you've finished simmering it, and steep them for 20 minutes.

If you are *only* using aromatic herbs, follow these guidelines for making syrup: Reduce the water from 5 cups to $1\frac{1}{2}$ cups and steep your herbs for 20 minutes. Strain and compost them, and then add the sweet syrup base and optional essential oils.

☀Basic Syrup

Use the amounts below for each cup of finished syrup; you can double or triple the recipe.

> 1–1½ cups fresh or ½–⅔ cup dried herbs
>
> 5 cups purified water
>
> 1 cup of a sweet syrup base, such as dehydrated cane juice, sugar, or honey (see page 163)
>
> Essential oils (optional)
>
> ½–1 level teaspoon vitamin C powder or ⅓ cup alcohol (optional, to preserve)

Blend or process the herbs to a coarse or fine consistency. Combine the herbs with the water in a saucepan, stir, and gently simmer, uncovered, for 20 minutes.

Turn off the heat and let the mixture steep for 20 minutes longer. Strain and compost the herbs. Pour the liquid back into the pan. Simmer and reduce the heat, and gently simmer, uncovered, until the liquid is reduced to about 1 cup. (If you're using sugar, add it halfway through the reducing process to make sure that it dissolves and thickens properly.) Let the mixture cool until warm, and add the sweet syrup base. Add a few drops of the optional essential oils and vitamin C powder or alcohol. Bottle, label, and store.

☀Garlic Syrup

An excellent way to take garlic as an antibiotic preventative when a cold is coming on.

> 2–5 cloves garlic
>
> 1 cup sweet syrup base (see page 163)
>
> 5 drops oregano essential oil (optional, for an antibacterial boost) or 2 or 3 drops peppermint or orange essential oil (for a flavor lift)

In a blender or food processor, combine the garlic, sweet syrup base, and essential oil. Blend or process until creamy. Bottle, label, and store.

☀Cough Syrup

This tasty syrup coats your throat, reduces irritation, and calms a persistent cough.

> 3–4 teaspoons fresh or 1½ teaspoons dried echinacea leaf, flower, and/or root
>
> 1½–2 teaspoons fresh or ¾ teaspoon dried licorice root
>
> 2 heaping teaspoons fresh or 1 teaspoon dried marshmallow root
>
> 3–4 teaspoons fresh or 1½ teaspoons dried orange peel
>
> 1½–2 teaspoons fresh or ¾ teaspoon dried sage leaf
>
> 3–4 teaspoons fresh or 1½ teaspoons dried thyme herb
>
> 5 cups purified water
>
> 1 cup sweet syrup base (see page 163)

Optional ingredients

> 2–3 teaspoons fresh or 1 teaspoon dried wild cherry bark (*Prunus serotina*)
>
> 3–4 teaspoons fresh or 1½ teaspoons dried horehound leaf (*Marrubium vulgare*; this herb adds extra cough-reducing power, but also has a bitter taste)
>
> 7 drops orange essential oil
>
> 3 drops peppermint essential oil
>
> Pinch of stevia per cup of finished liquid (optional, for sweetness)

If you're using fresh herbs, whir them in a blender, and if you're using dried, grind the herbs to a coarse or fine consistency. In a saucepan, simmer the echinacea, licorice, marshmallow, orange peel, and optional cherry bark in the water, uncovered, for 20 minutes. Turn off the heat. Add the sage, thyme, and optional horehound. Steep the entire mixture for 20 minutes longer, then strain and compost the herbs. Pour the liquid back into the saucepan, return it to a boil, reduce the heat, and gently simmer, uncovered, until the liquid is reduced to about 1 cup. Let it cool until it's warm and add the sweet syrup base and the optional essential oils. Stir well, bottle, label, and store.

Tinctures

Just as you can make a tea and extract your herb's medicinal constituents with hot water, you can do the same with a cool liquid—alcohol. You can grind and soak your fresh or dried herbs in an alcoholic liquid or solvent (such as vodka), then strain out the herbs. The resulting liquid is called a tincture.

Alcohol is an excellent solvent (meaning that the medicinal constituents of herbs dissolve in it very well). In our opinion, alcohol is second only to water! For most herbs, a hot tea will make the best herbal preparation, but in a few cases, tinctures can be an excellent choice.

Why make a tincture instead of a tea? Well, one reason is that alcohol will pull out the active constituents of the herbs as a cool liquid instead of as a hot one, which will better protect certain delicate constituents that can be boiled or steamed away by hot water (such as the oils that contribute to peppermint's lovely scent, or valerian's heat-sensitive active compounds). Alcohol carries the healing components of the herbs into your bloodstream quickly when you drink a tincture. In addition, alcohol is a very good preservative, so tinctures stored away from heat and light remain medicinally active for a year or more (and, depending on the herb, can sometimes remain viable for 2 to 3 years or longer). Tinctures are also portable and convenient—you can carry a small bottle with you and take it directly by mouth or by adding a few droppersful to water.

Tinctures are made by grinding or finely chopping up fresh or dried herbs, adding them to a solution of alcohol, letting the mixture stand for 2 to 3 weeks, and straining out the herbs. It's that simple!

You'll need to pay attention to the strength of your alcohol, because different herbs extract somewhat differently. Alcohol's strength is known as its "proof," and proof is written as twice the percentage of alcohol in the liquid. Some herbs need a higher proof alcohol to extract all of their medicinal constituents, while other herbs will yield their components better when the level of pure alcohol is lower. If the herb you want to tincture needs a very high alcoholic percentage, you'll need to use a higher proof alcohol; for other herbs, you can use a spirit with a lower level of pure alcohol, or you can dilute a high-proof alcohol with water to change its strength. (See page 210.) When you are making a tincture, the alcoholic liquid is technically called the "menstruum," and the herb, when you strain it out at the end, is called the "marc."

Finding the Right Solution

To obtain the correct level of alcohol for a menstruum, you have several choices. You can make your tincture with 100-proof vodka (50 percent pure alcohol), 160-proof vodka (80 percent pure alcohol), or 190-proof pure ethyl alcohol (95 percent pure alcohol). Ethyl alcohol is the strongest alcohol you can purchase, but it is restricted in some states; if you can obtain it, pure ethyl alcohol is often superior to vodka as a solvent. Traditionally, brandy has been used as a menstruum (it is 40 percent alcohol by volume), but modern brandy may contain pigments, flavoring compounds, sugars, and other components that diminish its ability to draw out the medicinal components of the herbs. We recommend using vodka or pure ethyl alcohol when available.

✳ Basic Tincture

A basic tincture is made with an herb (by weight, given in ounces), and a menstruum (by volume, given in liquid ounces). This recipe will make a little more than ½ cup of finished tincture.

> 2–3 ounces ground or finely chopped fresh or 1 ounce dried flowers, leaves, bark, seeds, or roots
>
> 5 liquid ounces vodka or ethyl alcohol

In a clean glass jar with a lid, combine the herb and the alcohol, making sure that the herb is completely submerged in the menstruum. If it's not, add more alcohol until the herb is completely covered by about 1 inch of liquid. Many herbalists recommend whirring the herb and the alcohol in a blender or food processor until pureed to make sure that lots of surface area is exposed on the herb. Cover the jar and store it in a dark place, shaking it daily for 2 to 3 weeks. Do not allow the herb to float above the level of the alcohol or the tincture will spoil; add more alcohol if necessary to keep the herb submerged. When the tincture is finished, filter it through cheesecloth, a coffee filter, or a fine-mesh strainer. Then put the herbs into a muslin bag, square of cheesecloth, or even a length of clean hosiery, draw the sides together, and squeeze out the last drops of liquid from the herbs. (You can even buy special herb presses that do the job well.) Compost the herb, pour the tincture into amber bottles, label the bottles with the contents and date, and store. Follow the dosage directions on page 210, or consult an experienced practitioner.

✳ Echinacea Tincture

You can take this tincture when you feel a cold coming on, or if you're treating an infection.

> 12 tablespoons fresh or 6 tablespoons dried ground or finely chopped echinacea root
>
> 2 cups 160-proof vodka (if using fresh herbs) or 100-proof vodka (if using dried herbs)

In a blender or food processor, combine the echinacea and alcohol. Blend or process until pureed. Pour the liquid into a clean glass jar with a lid, making sure that when it settles, the herb is completely submerged in the menstruum. If it's not, add more alcohol until the herb is covered by about 1 inch of liquid. Cover the jar and store it in a dark place, shaking it daily, for 2 to 3 weeks. Add more alcohol if necessary to keep the herb submerged. When the tincture is finished, filter it and then squeeze out the last drops of liquid from the herbs. Compost the herb, pour the tincture into amber bottles, label the bottles with the contents and date, and store.

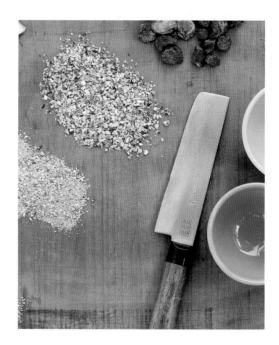

Oils

Herbal oils are simply oils infused with herbs, much as you'd steep rosemary in olive oil for culinary purposes. Healing herbal oils can be taken internally for a variety of ailments, can be used externally for therapeutic or daily beauty routines, and can be incorporated into herbal salve recipes. Dried herbs are preferred since fresh herbs will sometimes ferment.

Basic Herbal Oil

1 cup finely ground dried herbs (flowers, leaves, roots, barks, and/or seeds)

1¼ cups almond, jojoba, or olive oil

In a blender or food processor, combine the herbs and oil. Blend or process until pureed for greater extractability. Pour the mixture into a clean glass jar with a lid, making sure the plant material is completely submerged in the oil. If it's not, add more oil until the herbs are covered by about 1 inch of liquid. Cover the jar and store it in a dark place, shaking it daily, for 2 to 3 weeks. Filter it carefully through cheesecloth, a muslin bag, or a square of linen, gathering up the edges and squeezing out the oil. Compost the herbs. Pour the oil into amber bottles, and label the bottles with the contents and date. Store it in a dark place.

What Is an Essential Oil?

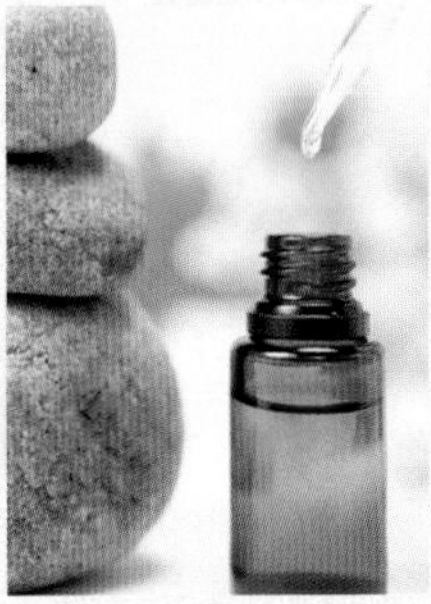

An essential oil is a highly concentrated compound, extracted from an herb, which gives the herb its characteristic fragrance. It is volatile, which means that it is easily dispersed in the air (think fragrance!) and can be distilled off and captured to produce a concentrated oil. It takes a large amount of herb to yield a small amount of oil, which accounts for the high price of commercially available essential oils. They are extremely concentrated—so strong that some are toxic—and should never be taken internally without professional advice. For external use, you should dilute an essential oil with a fixed oil, such as olive or almond, in order to avoid irritating your skin. When used safely and sparingly, essential oils add a delightful aroma and flavor to herbal preparations such as dried teas, tinctures, and salves.

☀Quick Infused Oil

Use this recipe when you need an herbal oil fast!

> 2 cups dried herbs (flowers, leaves, roots, barks, and/or seeds)
>
> 2 to 2½ cups almond, jojoba, or olive oil

In a blender or food processor, combine the herbs and oil. Blend or process until pureed. Place the mixture in a slow cooker turned to the low setting (about 100°F) and keep it covered. To prevent spoilage, keep the herb submerged in oil at all times; add more oil if necessary. Stir daily for about 3 days. Let the oil cool. Using a fine-mesh strainer or cloth, filter the herb out of the oil, pressing as much oil out as possible. Pour the oil into amber bottles, and label the bottles with the contents and date. Store it in a dark place.

☀St. John's Wort–Infused Oil

St. John's wort infused oil helps heal damaged nerves as well as other tissues. Conscientious, regular massage of an injured area with this oil can bring astonishing healing, even to old injuries. Taken internally, it helps heal stomach ulcers.

> 1 cup fresh St. John's wort flowering tops
>
> 1¼ cups almond, jojoba, or olive oil

In a blender or food processor, combine the herb and oil. Blend or process until smooth. Pour the mixture into a clean, clear glass jar and cover. Make sure the herb is submerged in the oil at all times; if necessary, add more oil. This oil should become bright red as it develops; if it does not, place the jar on a sunny windowsill where sunlight can warm it. Shake the jar vigorously every day for 2 to 3 weeks. Using a fine-mesh strainer or cloth, filter the herb out of the oil, pressing as much oil out as possible. Compost the herb, bottle and label the oil, and store it away from heat and light.

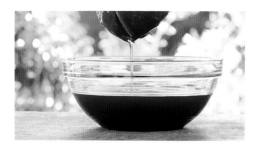

☀Earache Oil

This classic formula is a must for every family medicine chest and first-aid kit. It combines the properties of mullein flowers and garlic to reduce bacterial growth and prevent and ease earaches, wax buildup, and irritation. Remember, though, that ear infections, whether in children or adults, should be evaluated by a qualified healthcare practitioner before you treat them at home.

> 2 or 3 fresh garlic cloves
>
> 2 tablespoons fresh or dried mullein flower
>
> ½ cup almond, jojoba, or olive oil

Crush the garlic well and break up the mullein flower. In a blender or food processor, combine the garlic, flower, and oil. Blend or process until pureed. Pour the mixture into a clean, clear, glass pint jar and store it away from heat and light. Make sure the herb is submerged in the oil at all times; if necessary, add more oil. Shake the jar daily for about 2 weeks. Strain and compost the herb. Bottle and label the oil and store it away from heat and light.

To use, pour some oil into an amber bottle with a dropper, let it warm to room temperature, and put 2 or 3 drops of the oil into the ear that needs treatment. Tilt your head so the oil flows easily down your ear canal. Massage the back of your ear several times to help disperse the oil throughout the ear canal. Repeat two or three times daily.

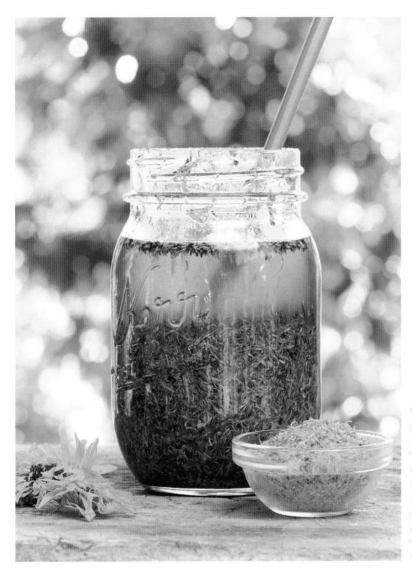

Calendula is a golden glory early in the summer and then throughout the summer and even fall in warmer climates. The flowering heads made into oils, salves, and creams are a centuries-old favorite for healing wounds and burns.

❋ Calendula Infused Oil

Apply this beautiful golden-colored oil directly to your skin to soothe rashes, sunburns, and skin irritations, or use it as part of a healing herbal salve or cream recipe. Store for up to 2 years if kept out of light and in a cool place.

> 1 cup wilted fresh or ½ cup dried calendula flowers
>
> 1¼ cups almond, jojoba, or olive oil

In a blender or food processor, combine the flowers and oil. Blend or process until pureed. Pour the mixture into a clean, clear glass jar, cover, and place in a warm spot out of direct sunlight. Make sure the herb is submerged in the oil at all times; if necessary, add more oil. Shake the jar vigorously every day for 2 to 3 weeks. Using a fine-mesh strainer or cloth, filter the herb out of the oil, pressing as much oil out as possible, and compost the herb. Bottle and label the oil and store it away from heat and light.

Compresses

Compresses are pads or cloths saturated with herbal teas that are then applied externally to heal skin traumas (wounds, rashes, skin infections, burns, scrapes, bites, and stings), contusions, sprains, strains, muscle aches, and even organ congestion (a lack of proper blood flow that can lead to the low functioning of an organ). A warm compress is helpful for aches and infections, while a cool compress soothes itching or burning pain. You can keep a warm compress heated with a hot water bottle and a cool compress chilled with an ice pack wrapped in a towel.

Warm compresses have a wide variety of healing uses: Calendula tea in a warm compress helps heal wounds and varicose ulcers, rosemary tea in a warm compress helps relieve the pain of arthritis or sore muscles, and thyme tea in a warm compress will prevent or relieve surface infections. Cool compresses reduce heat and soothe: Chamomile tea in a cool compress eases the pain of sunburn or rashes, and lemon balm tea can be used as an antiviral compress and applied to chicken pox and other herpes outbreaks. You can make a compress from any absorbent material—muslin, flannel, towels, and even old T-shirts. We use washcloths because they are absorbent by nature and are often a convenient size to use.

Apply a compress for healing and restoring the skin and relieving inflammation in the joints and muscles.

Basic Compress

Fold a soft cloth, saturate with a strong herb tea, and apply it to an area of the body in need of healing care—such as a bruise, strain, sprain, or inflammatory condition like an arthritic joint.

1. Cut a piece of muslin, flannel, toweling, or washcloth and fold it, if necessary, until it's slightly larger than the affected area.

2. Make a strong, dark tea by steeping 1 cup fresh or ½ cup dried herbs in 4 cups of purified water for about 20 minutes. If you're preparing a warm compress, the tea is ready to apply to the affected area. If you're preparing a cool compress, let the liquid cool.

3. Soak the compress cloth in the tea. Remove the cloth from the liquid, letting it drip and squeezing lightly until it is thoroughly wet but not dripping.

4. Apply the compress to the affected area. When a warm compress cools, reheat the liquid and renew the compress by dipping it into the liquid again. When a cool compress begins to feel dry or stiff, renew it by dipping it into the liquid again. You can also use a hot water bottle or ice pack.

5. You can use the same liquid for 2 days or you can make a fresh batch for each application. When reusing the same liquid, you may wish to bring the liquid to a boil first, to kill any bacteria, and then turn off the heat and let it cool to the desired temperature.

☀ "Eye" Love Herbs Compress

This traditional formula can soothe red, irritated eyes and reduce the inflammation and infection of pinkeye and styes. Oregon grape has a broad-spectrum antibacterial and antifungal effect, helping to reduce inflammation and irritation; eyebright is a traditional soothing herb for the eyes but can't be cultivated, so you'll need to purchase it or substitute the herbs we suggest for the same action. Use this tea as a compress, as a rinse in an eyecup, or by dropping a few drops into your eye from a dropper bottle, blinking to spread the liquid.

2 teaspoons fresh or 1 teaspoon dried Oregon grape stems or root

2 tablespoons fresh or 1 tablespoon dried eyebright (*Euphrasia officinalis*) herb, chamomile or mullein flowers, or lemon balm herb

½ cup purified water

Cotton balls or pads

Combine the Oregon grape and eyebright, chamomile, mullein, or lemon balm and water in a saucepan. Stir to thoroughly combine. Cover and bring it to a boil. Remove from the heat and steep for 10 minutes. Strain and compost the herbs. Soak a sterile cotton ball or pad in the tea, remove and gently squeeze the pad until it's wet but not dripping, and cover the infected eye. Tape the compress in place, if desired, or cover it with a small piece of plastic wrap, and cover all of that with a small washcloth. Keep it in place for 15 minutes. Reapply two or three times a day or as needed.

You can also use the cool tea in an eyecup two or three times a day. Fill the eyecup half full with the tea. Tilt your head forward over the eyecup, centering your eye socket over the rim and pressing against the socket to create a seal. With your eye open, tilt your head backward, blink, and roll your eye in a circular motion to allow the tea to rinse your entire eye. Keep the eyecup in place until you lower your head forward, to avoid spilling any tea. Discard the tea and rinse the eyecup well. Note: Remove contact lenses before using an eyewash.

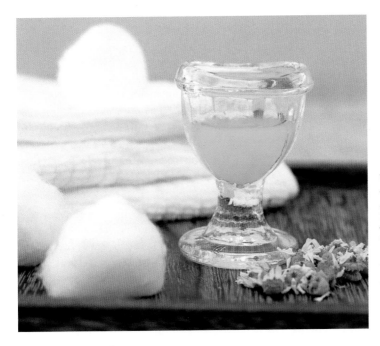

We love glass eyecups for their stability, but you'll find plastic ones just as effective. Eyecups are available in most pharmacies, or order them online. An herbal eye rinse can promote eye wellness, counteracting redness, itching, and dryness.

❋ Rash Compress

The herbs in this formula are astringent, soothing, and healing. Use it for poison ivy and oak, hives, blackheads, and acne that does not come to a head for draining.

½ cup fresh or ¼ cup dried calendula flowers

½ cup fresh or ¼ cup dried yarrow leaf

½ cup fresh or ¼ cup dried gotu kola leaf

½ cup fresh or ¼ cup dried self-heal or peppermint herb

4 cups purified water

2 or 3 drops peppermint essential oil (optional; use for hot, itchy rashes like poison oak and poison ivy)

Washcloth, muslin, or other absorbent cloth

Combine the calendula, yarrow, gotu kola, self-heal or peppermint, and water in a covered saucepan. Stir thoroughly to combine. Bring it to a boil, reduce the heat, and gently simmer for about 20 minutes. Let it cool and strain out the herbs, but do not discard them. Add the optional peppermint essential oil, and stir to mix well. Lay your washcloth or other compress cloth in a bowl and ladle about ¼ cup or more of the wet herbs, plus some of the tea, into the cloth. Gather the edges of the cloth around the herbs and secure with a tie, or hold the bundle closed.

Apply the herb compress to the affected area for 10 to 15 minutes. Return the bundle of herbs to the tea to soak for a few minutes, and apply the compress to the affected area again. Repeat one more time, for a total of three applications. Repeat this process two or three times daily, or as needed. You can also strain out the herbs, compost them, and just use the tea to soak your cloth (see Basic Compress on page 170).

Note: You can also apply St. John's wort infused oil, calendula oil or cream, or aloe vera gel to your skin between compress sessions; add a few drops of peppermint oil to these oils as well to cool hot, itchy rashes.

❋ Ginger Compress

This compress will help to relieve muscular or joint aches and pains, as well as speed healing and reduce the pain of injuries like strains or sprains. Ginger has a natural anti-inflammatory effect that reduces pain and swelling while increasing your circulation and the distribution of healing immune cells. Apply a ginger compress several times daily after you've used an ice-cold compress for 12 to 24 hours, as is usually medically recommended.

1 ounce fresh or ½ ounce dried ginger root

4 cups purified water

Washcloth, muslin, or other absorbent cloth

Combine the ginger and water in a saucepan, and stir to thoroughly combine. Bring to a boil, and gently simmer for 30 minutes. Sip ½ teaspoon of the ginger tea before you let it cool down; it should taste very spicy. If it doesn't, add another ounce of fresh ginger (or ½ ounce dried) to the tea and let it simmer for an additional 10 minutes before cooling. (Ginger can vary in its spiciness.)

Let the mixture cool to a temperature that is hot, but tolerable. Fold a washcloth or other compress cloth until it's slightly larger than the affected area, and dip it into the hot tea. Remove and squeeze gently, until the cloth is thoroughly wet but not dripping, and apply it to the injured area. Cover with a small plastic bag or plastic wrap (to prevent water loss) and then a small towel to keep in the heat; leave in place for 20 to 30 minutes.

You will feel the ginger compress cool down, but after about 20 minutes, you should feel it warming up again. This secondary feeling of warmth is due to the stimulating effect of the ginger itself. Leave the compress in place for 5 to 10 minutes after you feel this effect. Repeat the compress two or three times a day or as needed.

Creams, Lotions, and Salves

Dry, itchy skin? Cuts, scrapes, infected wounds, or rashes? They can all be soothed and renewed with the healing nourishment of herbs applied in a moisturizing base—the realm of creams, lotions, and salves. Of course, your skin is your largest eliminative organ. It's often exposed to the elements, and it's somewhat delicate (no fur or scales to protect it!). This means that it can take a beating from the weather and can be prone to wrinkling and drying. Because your skin breathes and eliminates toxins and other substances from your body, you may experience conditions such as rashes, acne, or boils as your skin releases these substances.

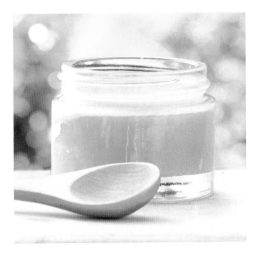

Creams, lotions, and salves are all marvelous ways to apply healing herbs to thirsty, damaged, or troubled skin, but they're each formulated slightly differently.

Cream. A cream is a mixture of oil and water, with a little wax added for body and texture. It's a bit like mayonnaise because it's an oil combined with a watery or nonoily substance whipped together so they don't separate (a process called emulsification). With mayonnaise, oil and eggs are mixed, while with a cream, oil and tea concentrates are combined. Many commercial creams include an emulsifier such as borax, which prevents the oil and water from separating, or they include substances that add texture, such as lanolin, cocoa butter, or acetyl alcohol. Our recipes also contain vitamin C powder, which acts as a mild preservative, but you can substitute an equal amount of ascorbic acid, which is available over the counter at pharmacies or in the canning area of the grocery store. Or you can add 2 or 3 drops of vitamin E or rosemary oil to the oil phase as a preservative. A cream moisturizes and soothes your skin.

Lotion. A lotion is similar to a cream, but it is lighter and contains more liquid. You can pour a lotion and spread it easily, which can really make a difference when you have inflamed, needy skin. By varying the ingredients, you can create lotions that are astringent, moisturizing, antifungal, antibacterial, or regenerative. Our lotions also contain vitamin C powder, as a preservative, and you can substitute vitamin E or rosemary oil just as you might in a cream.

Salve. A salve is a wonderful way to use your infused oils. Salves are made of oils and wax and are typically somewhat solid, so they're more convenient to use than oils. Although not as moisturizing as creams and lotions, salves last longer and provide a protective barrier that keeps bacteria out and moisture in. (Studies show that moist wounds heal faster than dry ones.) Salves keep the healing power of the herbs close to skin injuries, reducing inflammation and soreness and reducing cracked skin on feet and lips. Lip balms are a form of salve. Salves can be made with a single infused oil or with a combination of several; customizing a salve for individual use is part of the challenge and fun of making it.

On the following pages, you'll find a basic recipe for a cream, a lotion, and a salve, and then some sample recipes for you to try, using herbs from your garden. Be extra careful to wash all utensils, surfaces, containers, and your hands before beginning to make any of these recipes because this combination of ingredients is susceptible to spoilage. Keeping everything as hygienic as possible will yield long-lasting remedies.

If you make creams, please be aware that they spoil easily, so store them in your refrigerator if you're going to keep them for more than a few days. Don't introduce bacteria by dipping your fingers into the cream; instead, use a little craft stick or a small spoon to scoop it out of the jar.

✳ Basic Cream

Creams are composed mainly of oil and water, and each oil and water mixture is referred to as a "phase." The two phases are prepared and heated separately and then mixed together in a blender. You'll heat the two phases so they are as close as possible to the same temperature (160° to 175°F) before you combine them.

An emulsifier is required to hold the phases together in a creamy state. We use ordinary household borax as an emulsifier because it's a natural, gentle substance that does the job.

Oil Phase

½ ounce (2–3 teaspoons) beeswax

1 tablespoon coconut oil

4 tablespoons infused herbal oil

10–20 drops essential oil or combination of essential oils of your choice (optional, for fragrance or additional healing properties)

Water Phase

4 tablespoons tea concentrate (as you'd make for a dried tea) or strong tea infusion*

2 tablespoons aloe gel

½ –1 teaspoon borax

1 teaspoon vitamin C powder

Heat the beeswax, coconut oil, and infused herbal oil in a saucepan over medium heat until warm to the touch, but not hot. Add the optional essential oil. In another pan, heat the tea, aloe gel, borax, and vitamin C powder over medium heat until warm to the touch, but not hot. (Both phases should be heated to 160° to 175°F.)

Place the water phase ingredients in a blender and set it on high. Through the opening in the blender-jar cap, dribble in the oil phase ingredients. When the cream is thoroughly mixed, pour it into jars. Let it cool, cap the jars, label, and refrigerate.

*To make a strong tea infusion, combine 1 cup ground dried herbs and 1 cup freshly boiled water, and steep for 30 minutes, covered.

❋ Ginger-Cayenne Heat-Treatment Cream

Here's help for muscle aches and pains. You can make the infused oil yourself, using the recipe on page 167, with ½ cup ground or powdered dried ginger and ½ cup ground or powdered dried cayenne.

Oil Phase

½ ounce (2–3 teaspoons) beeswax

1 tablespoon coconut oil

4 tablespoons cayenne and ginger–infused oil

10–15 drops wintergreen essential oil (optional, for fragrance and pain-relieving activity)

Water Phase

4 tablespoons ginger tea concentrate (as you'd make for a dried tea)

2 tablespoons aloe gel

½ –1 teaspoon borax

1 teaspoon vitamin C powder

Heat the beeswax, coconut oil, and cayenne and ginger–infused oil in a saucepan over medium heat until warm to the touch, but not hot. Add the optional wintergreen essential oil. In another pan, heat the tea concentrate, aloe gel, borax, and vitamin C over medium heat until warm to the touch, but not hot. (Both phases should be heated to 160° to 175°F.)

Place the water phase ingredients in a blender and set it on high. Through the opening in the blender-jar cap, dribble in the oil phase ingredients. When the cream is thoroughly mixed, pour it into jars. Let it cool, cap the jars, label, and refrigerate.

❋ Skin Protection Cream

This cream prevents drying and chapping. It's formulated with glycerin, which is moisturizing and texturizing, making it lighter and extra creamy.

Oil Phase

1 ounce (about 1½ tablespoons) beeswax

2 tablespoons coconut oil

4 ounces almond oil

10–20 drops essential oil of your choice (for fragrance)*

Water Phase

2 ounces lemon balm, rosemary, or lavender strong tea infusion

2 ounces glycerin

1 teaspoon borax

1 teaspoon vitamin C powder

Heat the beeswax, coconut oil, and almond oil in a saucepan over medium heat until warm to the touch, but not hot. Add the essential oil. In another pan, heat the tea, glycerin, borax, and vitamin C powder over medium heat until warm to the touch, but not hot. (Both phases should be heated to 160° to 175°F.)

Place the water phase ingredients in a blender and set it on high. Through the opening in the blender-jar cap, dribble in the oil phase ingredients. When the cream is thoroughly mixed, pour it into jars. Let it cool, cap the jars, label, and refrigerate.

*For a sweet-smelling cream, try adding equal amounts of orange, grapefruit, lemon, and lavender essential oils to the basic cream. For an antiseptic cream to heal cuts and infections, stir in thyme, oregano, or tea tree essential oils. For a skin-protecting and age-defying cream, add rosemary essential oil and/or vitamin E oil (and use gotu kola tea for the water phase).

☀ Antifungal Cream

Use this handy cream for athlete's foot, ringworm, and other common fungal infections. Prevention is the best medicine here. Don't let an athlete's foot fungus migrate into your nails, where it can be very difficult or impossible to treat.

Oil Phase

½ ounce (about 2–3 teaspoons) beeswax

½ ounce (1 tablespoon) coconut oil

4 tablespoons calendula infused oil

10–20 drops oregano or thyme essential oil

Water Phase

4 tablespoons strong thyme tea infusion*

2 tablespoons aloe gel

½ –1 teaspoon borax

1 teaspoon vitamin C powder

Heat the beeswax, coconut oil, and calendula infused oil in a saucepan over medium heat until warm to the touch, but not hot. Add the essential oil. In another pan, heat the tea, aloe gel, borax, and vitamin C powder over medium heat until warm to the touch, but not hot. (Both phases should be heated to 160° to 175°F.)

Place the water phase ingredients in a blender and set it on high. Through the opening in the blender-jar cap, dribble in the oil phase ingredients. When the cream is thoroughly mixed, pour it into jars. Let it cool, cap the jars, label, and refrigerate.

*To make a strong tea infusion, combine 1 cup ground dried herb and 1 cup freshly boiled water, and steep for 30 minutes, covered.

☀ Basic Lotion

Good choices for the strong tea infusion are calendula, chamomile, comfrey, ginger, lavender, Oregon grape, peppermint, plantain, and rosemary.

½ teaspoon salt

½ cup strong tea infusion*

Cosmetic clay (available from Mountain Rose Herbals; see page 218)

½ teaspoon vitamin C powder

25 drops essential oil or combination of oils of your choice (for fragrance)

In a small bowl, dissolve the salt in the tea. Stir in the cosmetic clay and vitamin C powder until the mixture is creamy. Add the essential oil and blend thoroughly. Bottle, label, and refrigerate.

*To make the infusion, combine 1 cup ground dried herbs and 1 cup freshly boiled water, and steep for 30 minutes, covered.

☀ Poison Ivy or Poison Oak Lotion

This lotion works quickly and thoroughly for anyone suffering the misery of poison ivy or oak, any rash or burn, and even for acne.

½ teaspoon salt

½ cup combination of plantain and/or calendula strong tea infusion* and/or aloe vera gel

Cosmetic clay (available from Mountain Rose Herbals; see page 220)

25 drops peppermint essential oil

½ teaspoon vitamin C powder

In a small bowl, dissolve the salt in the tea or aloe gel. Stir in the cosmetic clay and vitamin C powder until the mixture is creamy. Add the essential oil and blend thoroughly. Pour into bottles and cap, label, and refrigerate. Apply as needed to the affected area, avoiding your eyes and mucous membranes.

*To make the infusion, combine ½ cup dried herb and ½ cup freshly boiled water, and steep for 30 minutes, covered.

❄ Basic Salve

Good choices for the infused oil in this recipe include calendula, cayenne, ginger, peppermint, rosemary, St. John's wort, and turmeric (although turmeric can stain).

1 ounce beeswax

1 cup infused oil

5–10 drops essential oil or combination of oils of your choice (for fragrance or additional healing action)

Grate the beeswax into a small bowl. In a saucepan or double boiler, heat the infused oil gently to about 100°F. Add the grated beeswax slowly, stirring as it melts. Turn off the heat and let the mixture cool for a few minutes before you add the essential oils. Stir to thoroughly combine. Pour your salve into jars and let it cool. Cap and label the jars. Apply the salve as needed to the affected area. You can store a salve indefinitely.

❄ Healing Salve

Use to reduce inflammation and lessen the possibility of infection from a skin injury.

1 ounce beeswax

1 cup infused oil, using equal parts calendula, yarrow, and St. John's wort–infused oils

5–10 drops essential oils of your choice, such as lavender, orange, mint, or thyme (for fragrance)

Grate the beeswax into a small bowl. In a saucepan or double boiler, heat the infused oil gently to about 100°F. Add the grated beeswax slowly, stirring as it melts. Turn off the heat and let the mixture cool for a few minutes before you add the essential oils. Stir thoroughly to combine. Pour your salve into jars and let it cool. Cap and label the jars. Apply the salve as needed to the affected area. You can store a salve indefinitely.

Tips for Salves

If you prefer a salve that's harder or softer than this recipe, just add more or less beeswax or oil. You can test the consistency of the salve before it hardens by scooping out a spoonful and dipping the back of the spoon into a little bowl of ice water to harden the salve. If it's too soft for your taste, heat the ingredients again and add more beeswax. If it's too hard, heat the ingredients again and add a bit more oil. Test after each addition to get the consistency you prefer. Sometimes, after the salve is poured into a jar and when it's nearly set, a small crater will appear in the middle of the surface. You can add a small amount of hot salve to the crater to create an even surface.

❄ Healing Lip Balm

A lip balm is no different than a salve in its formulation, except that you may wish to make it a little firmer. This one works wonders for chapped, dry lips.

1 ounce beeswax

1 cup infused oil (calendula, ginger, peppermint or spearmint, rosemary, and St. John's wort are good choices)

5–10 drops essential oils of your choice (for fragrance)

Grate the beeswax into a small bowl. In a saucepan or double boiler, heat the infused oil gently to about 100°F. Add the grated beeswax slowly, stirring as it melts. Turn off the heat and let the mixture cool for a few minutes before you add the essential oils. Stir to thoroughly combine. Pour your mixture into lip balm tubes and let it cool. Cap and label the tubes.

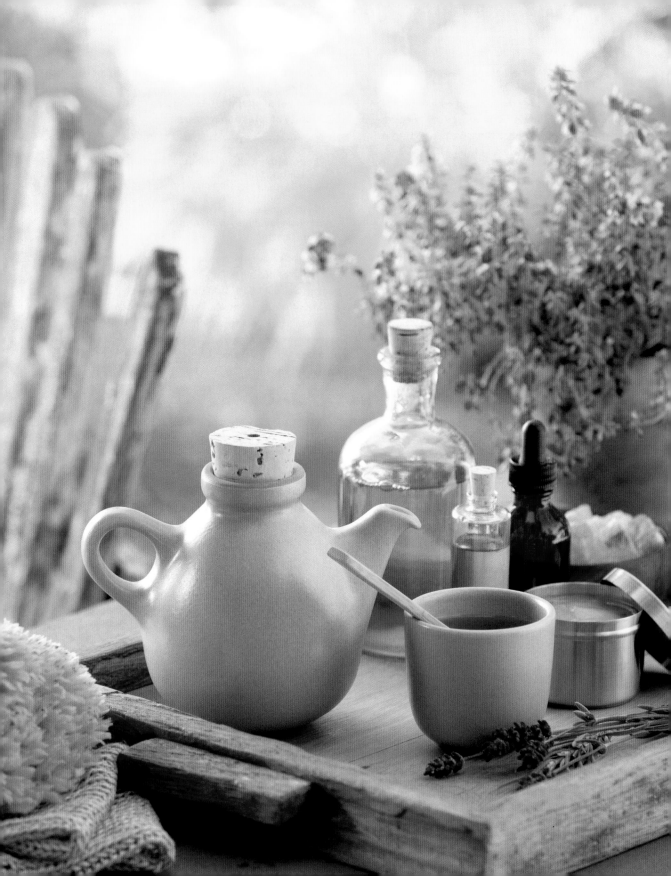

PART 4

Heal It

Time for healing! In this section, discover how to use herbs in practical terms—from dosage amounts to treatments and regimes. With an emphasis on prevention and without using complex medical terms, we present herbal remedies that offer relief and healing from a wide variety of symptoms and ailments. Most important of all, you can trust this advice: It's research-based and cites the experience of herbal practitioners and medical studies that show that herbs have been safely used to treat patient volunteers in thousands of clinical studies.

All of us want to live happy, fulfilling, and creative lives. How can we achieve that goal? Well, undoubtedly, creating and maintaining good health is key. **Most importantly, we need to pay attention to what is unfolding in and around us. This means regular internal "check-ins" to determine what we need—rest, nutrients, emotional and physical contact, stretching and movement—as well as the daily practice of healthy habits. We must literally *practice to be healthy* rather than practice to be sick. Like learning to play the piano or speak a new language, this requires effort, knowledge, support, and repetition. In today's world, it also necessitates knowing how best to manage the daily stress that is part of our lives in a way that works for us personally and individually.**

Reducing stress and its effect on health is a challenge for nearly everyone. Some of us turn to pharmaceutical medications, which often not only fail to truly reduce stress, but actually make our symptoms worse! We can become trapped in a cycle of experiencing stress, trying to treat the stress, and finding it escalating, rather than subsiding.

To break the pattern, you must step out of it and pursue alternatives, rebuild your vital energy, and practice methods and habits that bring true stress reduction. Just as we have developed habits of stress, we can now build habits of restorative health.

Although stress is an unavoidable part of contemporary life, there are natural ways of relieving it and preventing or treating its symptoms—approaches that are both ancient and proven. When exploring these methods, the first thing to remember is that all of the systems of your body require periods of rest and periods of activity in order to function well. It is the periods of rest that many of us find difficult to take, because the frenetic activities of our lives have become so habitual that they seem essential. However, if we don't have periods of revitalizing rest, we'll become ever more vulnerable to bouts of serious illness. Without health, all of the things that we're now working for so frantically will be difficult to enjoy.

Another very important activity is inner work—connecting with a higher wisdom or a spiritual path, resolving old hurts, reaching for understanding, asking forgiveness for wrongs, and forgiving others. If this aspect is ignored, we'll continually create turmoil in our lives, which can be the first and foremost source of stress.

The final pillar of any restorative regime is practical, daily attention to supporting our bodies' efforts to heal themselves and maintain health. We can do this by assuring ourselves adequate rest balanced with activity, by employing techniques that create peace and calm in our lives (such as meditation and yoga), and by using natural herbs and foods wisely and consciously.

Since ancient times, the majority of people in the world have used medicinal herbs to prevent disease and restore good health. Approximately 60 to 70 percent of people in the Third World, as well as 600 million Chinese, still rely on herbal medicine for their primary health care. However, until recently, the use of medicinal herbs in the United States had been largely supplanted by pharmaceutical drugs. But the fact that you've picked up this book and want to learn more is testimony to a wave of change taking place today. Due in part to concerns about the potential harm of prescription drugs and in part to a new awareness of health alternatives, interest in wellness-enhancing herbs is increasing rapidly.

In the pages ahead, you'll find profiles of some of the major health concerns you may be encountering, as well as ways that you can work toward solutions and healthy habits. We hope you will use this information to bring about the changes you need and to become more familiar with the extraordinary power of herbal medicine. Please remember that we're presenting the historical and modern record of the use of herbs to support your good health, but we are not prescribing herbs for any medical condition. Work with your doctor or health-care practitioner to incorporate herbal remedies into your existing treatment plan. A complete program of action, which includes the safe and proper use of herbs, is the only lasting and sure way to achieve and maintain vibrant health.

Arthritis and Sore Joints

Arthritis is a chronic inflammatory condition of your joints, associated with symptoms like redness, pain, swelling, stiffening, and finally degenerative changes in your joints and bones. It occurs in genetically susceptible individuals and is caused by chronic inflammation. Inflammation has recently been recognized and widely acknowledged in the medical community as an important underlying factor in many diseases.

What Helps: Chronic inflammation can arise from eating a diet high in red meat, refined sugar, spicy and fried foods, and stimulants like coffee, as well as from stress and overwork combined with poor sleep and exercise habits. Inflammation often takes many years to develop, so symptoms might not occur until you're in your 40s or 50s, or even later. Improving your eating patterns is crucial to reducing inflammation, and it's never too late to make a change. Many herbs and foods have natural anti-inflammatory properties, and you can use them on a daily basis to bring inflammation into a normal range, helping to relieve symptoms.

Herbs to Grow and Use: The following herbs can be taken as teas (infusions or decoctions), tinctures, or in capsule form unless otherwise noted below. You can make your own or purchase commercial inflammation-fighting dietary supplements containing these herbs. Some of them, such as hops and turmeric, are particularly well researched.

- Hops can help moderate inflammation when consumed in nonalcoholic or alcoholic beers. (However, please be aware that consumption of alcohol is counterproductive, and we recommend moderation.)

- Turmeric can be used liberally in cooking and teas.

- Licorice, ligustrum, and red clover are all pleasant-tasting anti-inflammatory agents.

Burns and Sunburns

First-degree burns damage the outer layer of your skin, causing pain, redness, and swelling. Second-degree burns affect the first two layers of your skin, causing blistering in addition to the pain, redness, and swelling of first-degree burns. Third-degree burns are the most serious and extend into deeper tissues. Third-degree burns, second-degree burns that cover an area more than 2 to 3 inches in diameter, or burns on your hands, feet, face, groin, buttocks, or a major joint are all serious medical emergencies and should be treated by a health-care professional right away.

What Helps: For first- and second-degree burns, immediately apply cold water or a cold or iced compress to the affected area, or soak it in water as cold as is comfortable for 5 to 10 minutes or more. Next, apply aloe vera gel or a healing herbal salve or cream (such as "Healing Salve" on page 177) to the area as often as possible during the day.

Herbs to Grow and Use: We particularly recommend applying the fresh gel and juice of aloe—which usually provides quick relief—and St. John's wort oil throughout the day. The following herbs can be taken as teas (infusions or decoctions), tinctures, or in capsule form unless otherwise noted below.

- Aloe vera is invaluable. Slice the leaf and squeeze out the gel. Keep a piece of fresh leaf in a small plastic bag in your pocket or purse when you're nursing a burn while you're away from home.

- St. John's wort or calendula oil, either homemade or purchased, can be applied liberally and frequently after treating a burn with cold or ice.

- Plantain leaf can be used in a poultice.

- Comfrey pulp is also soothing. Crush the roots and apply the slimy pulp directly or in a small cloth bag; change it when the pulp dries out.

Cholesterol Balance

High cholesterol, also called hyperlipidemia, is an excessive amount of cholesterol circulating in the blood and in body tissues. A high level is defined as a total cholesterol level above 200 mg/dl, or levels of high-density cholesterol (HDL, or so-called "good" cholesterol) below 35 mg/dl, or a ratio of HDL to low-density cholesterol (LDL, or so-called "bad" cholesterol) lower than 4:1. Cholesterol is produced by the liver, and high levels of cholesterol have been associated with increased risk of cardiovascular disease and early death. Causative factors include stress, a high intake of refined sugar or hydrogenated oil, regular consumption of animal fats, and genetics.

What Helps: A diet high in fruits, vegetables, and fiber, especially lots of whole grains and beans, can be helpful in lowering cholesterol. An herbal treatment will include a combination of herbs that help to lower high cholesterol and herbs that balance liver and bile functions.

Herbs to Grow and Use: Cooking frequently with garlic and turmeric can help add a tasty zest to your cholesterol-management efforts! Herbs such as artichoke leaf activate liver function and combine well in a "bitters" formula.

The following herbs can be taken as teas (infusions or decoctions), tinctures, or in capsule form unless otherwise noted below.

- Alfalfa is recommended by herbalists to maintain a healthy cholesterol balance.

- Aloe, commercially available as a diluted gel or juice, helps maintain normal bowel function.

- Artichoke helps promote bile flow and lowers cholesterol.

- Dandelion root can be taken as a healthy liver tea, or you can eat the stir-fried greens.

- Crushed garlic may be stirred into soups, stews, and other dishes. Raw garlic is always stronger-acting than cooked garlic.

- Cooking with turmeric helps maintain proper liver function to balance cholesterol.

Colds, Flu, and Respiratory Tract Infections

We all know about colds and flu, and only too well. The average person in the United States gets an average of 2.5 colds every year, and when you consider the total population (about 300 million people), that amounts to three-quarters of a billion colds per year. It's no wonder that pharmacies are stocked with remedies to help reduce the symptoms: headache, body aches, sore throat, nasal congestion, low energy, and poor sleep. Fortunately, you can grow and prepare many herbs that effectively counteract the symptoms of colds and flu.

What Helps: Sleep is one key to avoiding colds in the first place. Recent studies performed at UCLA showed that volunteers were much less likely to get sick when they had a good 8 hours of sleep per night, as compared to those who got less than 8 hours and those who didn't sleep well. Frequent hand washing is also known to reduce the incidence of upper respiratory tract infections that are viral in nature. Remember that many viral agents enter your body through the mucous membranes of your eyes: Touching an infected doorknob and then rubbing your eyes, for instance, can greatly increase your risk of becoming infected.

Herbs to Grow and Use: Herbs to help prevent and treat the symptoms of common colds, flus, and other respiratory tract infections fall into several categories. The following herbs can be taken as teas (infusions or decoctions), tinctures, or in capsule form, unless otherwise noted below.

- Immune-tonic herbs that help prevent infections include astragalus, garlic, ligustrum, and self-heal.

- Immune stimulants, which help activate defenses when the first symptoms occur, should be taken throughout an infection and finish up 4 to 5 days later to avoid rebound infections. These herbs include echinacea, garlic, lemon balm, oregano, thyme, and tulsi basil.

- Some herbs target specific cold and flu symptoms: Elder, peppermint, and yarrow reduce fever, sage helps calm a sore throat, and California poppy will ease headaches.

- Antiviral herbs to slow down the activity and spread of a virus include andrographis, elder (berry), thyme, and yerba mansa.

In practice, the functions of many of these herbs overlap. Echinacea, for instance, can help relieve a number of symptoms associated with respiratory tract infections.

Constipation and Regulation of Bowels

Go into any pharmacy and look for the aisle that holds the laxatives. It's usually full of a diverse array of products to help with regularity. These often contain the powerful stimulant laxative senna (*Senna alexandrina*) or the bulk laxative psyllium seed and husk (*Plantago ovata*).

Constipation is the result of a number of factors, the primary one being a lack of fiber in your diet. We eat only about one-tenth of the fiber our ancestors consumed, which was mostly in the form of whole grains, legumes, fruits, wild greens, and roots. Fiber is stimulating to the bowels and helps to remove wastes and regulate cholesterol. It also feeds beneficial bacteria that produce nutrients (such as B vitamins) and activate and strengthen our immune processes.

Other conditions that contribute to constipation include excessive sitting, constant eating without taking pauses, overeating, drinking beverages containing stimulants, and regular consumption of highly refined foods.

What Helps: Frequently including fiber in your diet, in any form—beans, whole grains, vegetables, or fruits—can help considerably. Exercise will keep things moving, as will adequate fluids, and most fresh fruits and veggies will help hydrate the bowels.

Self-massage of the abdominal area with a little St. John's wort oil, or even through your clothes, without the oil, can help relax and remove the tension in your abdominal area, resulting in better bowel movements.

Herbs to Grow and Use: The following herbs can be taken as teas (infusions or decoctions), tinctures, or in capsule form unless otherwise noted below.

- Aloe gel, although mild, does act as a bowel stimulant when consumed several times a day.

- Bitter herbs that activate the bile flow from the liver, as well as other digestive enzymes, can promote regularity. These include artichoke leaf, Oregon grape root, turmeric, and wormwood.

- Aromatic, warming herbs such as angelica and fennel promote good circulation to the bowels and increase the release of digestive enzymes.

- Marshmallow root is mucilaginous and soothing to the digestive tract, and it helps to reduce irritation in the gut.

Cough

Coughing is a protective mechanism for your body. When you have a respiratory tract infection like a cold, flu, pneumonia, or bronchitis, your throat is often irritated due to your body's immune response to the virus. The cough reflex helps clear your lungs and bronchial area of mucus laden with wastes from the battle against virally infected cells.

What Helps: Recent research has confirmed that sleep is one of the most important immune strengtheners available to us, and getting at least 8 hours each night, especially during stressful times and in the winter months, can help prevent the respiratory tract infections that commonly lead to coughs. Drinking warm or hot respiratory teas with immune-boosting properties can also help greatly. We recommend mullein and licorice tea with a little echinacea, for instance, as a daily brew, off and on, during the cold season.

Herbs to Grow and Use: The following are excellent herbs to help prevent coughs or reduce their severity. They can be taken as teas (infusions or decoctions), tinctures, or in capsule form unless otherwise noted below.

- Mullein can be used as a daily tea, sweetened with stevia or licorice.

- Licorice is a great expectorant; use it throughout the cold season.

- Sage is one of the very best sore throat and cough remedies. The leaves can be chewed and the juice swallowed to soothe a sore throat.

- Echinacea, perhaps blended with lemon balm, keeps your immune system active during the winter months.

- Marshmallow tea can be sipped to reduce throat irritation.

Dermatitis, Rashes, and Acne

Dermatitis is an inflammatory condition of the dermis, or skin, and it can arise from allergic reactions to foods or other allergens, such as pollen, or exposure to irritating chemicals in the environment, like harsh soaps or paint. Another common factor is chronic stress or pressure. It is important to identify the irritants and eliminate them, or to identify the source of stress and take steps to reduce or eliminate it.

What Helps: Your herbal program might include soothing and anti-inflammatory herbal creams and herbs taken internally to speed healing of your skin. If the condition is chronic, include digestive stimulants to increase stomach acid and other digestive enzymes, along with immune modulators (herbs that activate your body's immune system).

Herbs to Grow and Use: Some herbs can be used externally to provide local relief from inflammation and itching; you can make creams and compresses from the recipes in Make It (see page 143). Others can be consumed frequently to help balance the internal processes involved in chronic skin eruptions. The following herbs can be taken as teas (infusions or decoctions), tinctures, or in capsule form unless otherwise noted below.

- Calendula cream, or the tea as a warm compress, can be applied to irritated skin.

- Plantain, yarrow, and Oregon grape tea in a compress can soothe acne.

- Aloe gel can relieve itching and inflammation when applied directly to your skin.

- Chamomile tea will soothe a rash when applied as a cool compress.

- Elder (flower) tea can be drunk to reduce inflammation and to ease chronic skin eruptions.

- Red clover is a leading cleansing herb used to help reduce skin problems at the source.

- Burdock stimulates bile flow and liver function to help the liver process toxins.

Diabetes

Diabetes is a metabolic (meaning related to all the processes of digestion, assimilation, and energy production and utilization) disease that develops when the insulin in your body can't adequately move sugar out of your bloodstream and into your cells. Diabetes can develop from excessive and chronic intake of refined sugars along with severe, ongoing stress, or it can have a hereditary basis. In mild cases, supplemental insulin can be taken orally. In more severe cases, it must be injected daily.

What Helps: A diet low in fat and sugar and high in fiber is essential to preventing and managing diabetes, as is adequate exercise. An herbal program can include adaptogens (herbs that help your body adapt to external stressors and changes and help to balance your body's metabolic processes), herbs to help stabilize blood sugar and balance your metabolism, herbs that lower blood sugar, and pancreatic tonics.

Herbs to Grow and Use: While not curative, adding these herbs to your diet on a regular basis can support your efforts to maintain healthy blood sugar levels and insulin metabolism balance. The following herbs can be taken as teas (infusions or decoctions), tinctures, or in capsule form unless otherwise noted below.

- Love-in-a-mist has tasty seeds you can add to salads, soups, and other dishes.

- Aloe gel or juice can be used regularly in drinks and juices.

- Turmeric can be used frequently as a spice, and it's found in most curry dishes.

- Stevia can be used as a sweetener in drinks and cooking to help reduce your sugar intake (it's noncaloric!).

- Garlic, crushed, may be stirred into soups, stews, and other dishes. Raw garlic is always stronger-acting than cooked garlic.

Digestive Problems
(Dyspepsia, Pain, and Fullness After Eating)

Consider your digestion: It is responsible for supplying your body with all the energy it needs throughout the day, every day, from the moment you are born. Since about 60 percent of your immune tissues, as well as many billions of bacteria, live in your gut (the small and large intestines), your digestive tract is also vitally involved in your immune response. Finally, your digestive tract also produces a number of hormones, such as serotonin, that regulate your sleep response and mood (among many other functions). Considering all that your digestive tract is responsible for, it is truly the foundation of health.

When things go wrong, they can go wrong in a big way and can adversely affect your mood, energy level, strength, vitality, and immune response. Discomfort and pain in the abdominal area, constipation, gas, and diarrhea are only localized symptoms that signal an imbalance, but the impact of any digestive imbalance can be much wider and have few noticeable signs.

What Helps: One very healthy digestive habit is self-massage of your abdominal area daily—for up to 5 minutes. Lie on your back, move your hands in a clockwise fashion, and stroke deeply, working out any "stuck" or painful places. Keep it up, and you will notice direct results, including less gas and discomfort after eating.

Eat simply, and avoid overeating. Be careful at potluck meals: They are an opportunity to combine too many foods at once. Our digestive process prefers simple combinations of foods and prefers them not to be coated in oil or fried, which slows their assimilation and breakdown. Rest your digestion regularly by not eating too late at night or too early in the morning,

and by observing regular days of very light eating—only simple porridges, whole grains, raw foods, juices—or even fasting. The habit of under-calorizing can reset your system. Regular intake of probiotics ("friendly" bacteria that aid digestion, similar to the active cultures found in yogurt), in amounts between 20 and 50 billion organisms a day, can truly help regulate your bowels and improve digestion.

Foods that have no nutrients (doughnuts, white bread, soft drinks) take energy to process but give you little in return. Remember: If it has no nutritional value, don't eat it or drink it!

Herbs to Grow and Use: Herbalists recommend herbs for all aspects of digestive function and dysfunction, and those herbs can be placed in several categories. The following herbs can be taken as teas (infusions or decoctions), tinctures, or in capsule form unless otherwise noted below.

- Digestive stimulants help increase enzyme production, which brings vitality to the digestive processes and enhances assimilation. These include angelica, artichoke, cayenne (and other spicy peppers), garlic, ginger, turmeric, and wormwood. These herbs can be taken before eating or incorporated into a meal, as is common in many world cuisines.

- Carminatives help relieve gas and regulate digestion to keep things moving smoothly. This includes anise hyssop, basil, catnip, fennel, love-in-a-mist, oregano, peppermint, sage, and thyme. They can be consumed as a warm tea, right after a meal.

- Bowel-movers and regulators include aloe gel, burdock, Oregon grape root, and especially yellow dock (see page 105). Use these herbs regularly, before bedtime, to help produce better movements the next day.

- Herbs to settle the digestion and relieve discomfort and nausea include ginger, lavender, lemon balm, lemon verbena, peppermint, wormwood, and yarrow. These herbs can be used after meals if you experience discomfort.

Fatigue

Fatigue is a state that most of us know well. It's not always an unpleasant feeling, but when it becomes chronic, fatigue can be devastating. However, this condition should not be confused with the feeling of being pleasantly tired after a day of hiking or gardening, when you might look forward to relaxing in your favorite chair or getting a good night's sleep. Vigorous physical activity provides benefits for your cardiovascular system, helps to keep you fit and vital, slows the aging process, and helps you to sleep more soundly.

Have you ever had a feeling of heaviness in your arms and legs, a lack of vitality, poor mental clarity, and a lowered ambition or drive to accomplish your dreams? It's normal to experience these occasionally, but days or weeks of the same condition can be termed "chronic fatigue" and needs to be addressed.

Chronic fatigue, to one degree or another, is all too common today, as evidenced by the ever-increasing consumption of foods and drinks containing caffeine and high amounts of refined sugar. Soft drinks, energy drinks, coffee, and green tea are available at every grocery store, quick stop, home improvement outlet, and produce stand. Many of us need our "fix"—frequently, it seems—to get up and out in the morning, to keep going, and to counteract the feeling of tiredness that accompanies long hours at the computer.

Just as you manage your financial resources, you can also manage your energy resources. Think of caffeine and refined sugar as a credit card. When you run out of energy and feel tired, you can "borrow" more energy by stimulating your nervous system and hormones with these two energy boosters. But as we all know, that pattern cannot go on forever. A better "stimulus package" is a combination of natural medicine and healthy habits.

In this energy equation, remember to avoid consuming "empty calorie" foods (such as white flour products that provide no nutrients but take significant energy to process and eliminate), holding yourself tight in response to stress, worrying constantly, or getting worked up emotionally over trivial matters.

What Helps: There are a number of ways you can save and even increase your energy levels. These include stretching and yoga to release tension, a whole foods diet containing lots of fiber, and meditation. Also, consider that much of the tiredness you feel might not be from a lack of energy at all, but rather may be from a condition that traditional Chinese medicine calls "stagnation." When you sit too much, your body's processes are bogged down. Blood and energy pool in your muscles and organs and do not move vitalizing nutrients and oxygen or remove wastes.

We all know some celebrated herbs that help supply us with more energy: coffee and tea. These herbs stimulate your body's processes and increase mental functioning when you get bogged down, and they have been used in traditional societies for thousands of years. Green tea is the second most widely consumed drink in the world, and for good reason: You can get a "benefit with the buzz," because green tea has significant protective and healing benefits in addition to a moderate amount of caffeine. However, in our overly caffeinated society, there are other herbs that can help promote abundant energy, rather than just stimulating your nervous system and hormones.

Herbs to Grow and Use: The following herbs can be taken as teas (infusions or decoctions), tinctures, or in capsule form unless otherwise noted below.

- Angelica, artichoke, and fennel help to promote more complete digestion by activating enzymes from the liver and other digestive organs.

- Ashwagandha is recommended for counteracting stress and increasing energy.

- Astragalus activates immunity and counteracts fatigue when used regularly.

- Burdock is a regular part of the Japanese diet, and it's used to promote increased vitality.

- Chamomile and lavender are good-tasting herbs that encourage relaxation and release nervous tension.

- Rosemary contains several constituents, such as camphor, that help to vitalize your nervous system.

- Licorice and ligustrum are often recommended as adaptogens, which help to counteract the harmful effects of stress and increase energy.

- Love-in-a-mist promotes good digestion and energy.

- Rhodiola is widely taken in Russia and Scandinavia (and increasingly in other parts of the world) to increase stamina, support clear thinking, and counteract stress.

Fever

Fever can be a beneficial and normal part of your body's immune function, indicating that your immune system is on alert and helping you to fight bacterial and viral infections. Fevers are also associated with injuries and certain metabolic disorders, such as hyperthyroidism. Low, chronic fevers can be a symptom of ongoing mild inflammation, which is now thought to underlie most, if not all, chronic diseases like arthritis, diabetes, and heart disease.

What Helps: If the fever comes on quickly in response to a viral infection, you can take internal heat-clearing (cooling) herbs to manage it, along with herbs that contain natural salicylates (as are found in aspirin), like willow bark (*Salix alba*) tea (or a standardized extract) or meadow-sweet leaf (*Filipendula ulmaria*) tea. Internal heat can also be cleared through the urine with the help of cooling and diuretic herbs. When a fever gets too high (over 104°F), cool off with herbal sponge baths or even soak in a tub of cool water along with following your herbal regime, and check with your health professional.

Herbs to Grow and Use: The following herbs can be taken as teas (infusions or decoctions), tinctures, or in capsule form unless otherwise noted below.

- Catnip, elder (flower), echinacea, honeysuckle, lemon balm, peppermint, Oregon grape, self-heal, and yarrow are all great herbs to use as infusions and decoctions for fevers. You can take a cup or more every hour or two throughout the day to lower a fever. Make a blend of these herbs that tastes good to you in terms of strength and balance of the herb combination.

Gallbladder and Kidney Stones

Your gallbladder stores and concentrates the bile produced by your liver. Bile is essential for proper fat digestion and assimilation. It's important to keep bile production and movement at a healthy rate, as your body needs it. When it becomes "stagnant" (when you are experiencing poor fat digestion), liver and gallbladder ailments can result, as well as metabolic disorders related to improper fat metabolism.

What Helps: Use herbs to help keep your bile moving and your bile chemistry in proper balance. A supportive diet should be low in processed fats and high in daily servings of fiber, organic fruits, and green, leafy vegetables of all kinds (especially bitter ones like dandelion). Avoid too many spicy and greasy, fried foods.

Herbs to Grow and Use: The following herbs can be taken as teas (infusions or decoctions), tinctures, or in capsule form unless otherwise noted.

- Include dandelion (leaf and root) in your diet, and take artichoke and wormwood as teas and elixirs to promote a healthy production, flow, and balance of bile. You can also take capsules of these herbs, with the exception of wormwood, which is primarily used as a tea infusion.

Gas

Flatulence is abundantly produced in all mammals by bacterial action on food residues that reach the large intestine. It can be made in large quantities, and believe it or not, it is a main contributor to greenhouse gases and global warming. Millions of cows and other ruminants are responsible for enormous quantities of carbon dioxide (CO_2) gas released into the atmosphere worldwide. Gas produced by humans is not itself harmful, but it can be annoying and sometimes embarrassing. Excessive flatulence can be a sign of incomplete or weak digestion.

What Helps: Beans are a notorious source of gas. Make sure to soak dried beans overnight, and slow-cook them until they're very tender. (Undercooked beans, sometimes served in restaurants, are a problem for many people.) Take bitter tonics and add bitter greens (such as endive salad) to your diet, especially before eating fatty or protein-rich meals. And remember to eat slowly and chew well.

Herbs to Grow and Use: We recommend the following herbs to curb gas. They can be taken as teas (infusions or decoctions), tinctures, or in capsule form unless otherwise noted below.

- Dandelion greens can be added fresh to salads for a bitter taste or cooked for a milder therapeutic effect.

- Both wormwood and artichoke tea, taken before meals, help to keep bile moving and inhibit gas.

- Anise hyssop, fennel, or love-in-a-mist tea, when consumed after a meal, helps to inhibit excessive gas formation and reduce abdominal gas pains.

- Peppermint, in the form of tea or candy, is the last herbal holdout in many mainstream restaurants. And you can always carry a small bottle of peppermint oil in your pocket or purse; just add 2 or 3 drops to a cup of hot water with a lemon slice and sip that after your meal.

Headache

A headache is a common symptom that can signify many things: musculoskeletal tension in your neck and shoulders, eye strain, allergic reactions, temporary withdrawal from caffeine or other substances, stress and worry, and a host of other causes.

What Helps: Self-massage of your neck and shoulders, or better still, a loving massage from a partner or friend, can do wonders to relieve a headache, and very quickly. A walk in the fresh air while taking some deep, relaxing breaths, which gets your circulation moving and lets your mind wander, is a solution to some kinds of headaches, and a quiet period of rest and relaxation helps others. In the winter, a warm cup of herbal tea, and in the summer, a cool glass of herbal iced tea, can be healing and pleasant.

Herbs to Grow and Use: We recommend relaxing herbs, herbs to increase blood flow to your head, herbs to relieve liver stagnation, and cooling herbs. The following herbs can be taken as teas (infusions or decoctions), tinctures, or in capsule form unless otherwise noted below.

- California poppy, chamomile, lavender, and skullcap are antispasmodic and relaxing. Drink 1 cup of tea two or three times a day.

- Gotu kola and rosemary improve your circulation. Try a cup of tea two or three times daily.

- Lavender oil can be used as aromatherapy throughout the day, as a cream, or in a relaxing bath.

- Artichoke or burdock can regulate the liver, if this is part of the problem. Both herbs make refreshingly bitter teas.

Heart Health

Your heart is a tireless organ that beats throughout your life, so it pays to consider its health from time to time. Your heart and blood vessels work together, and over time, the vessels can stiffen and become clogged, increasing your risk of high blood pressure and heart disease. See "Hypertension" and "Cholesterol Balance" on pages 193 and 182 for more information about specific conditions affecting your heart.

What Helps: A simple, whole foods diet with very little added processed sugar and fat will be of great benefit to your heart. Lots of love and positive thoughts and deeds are certain to provide more than a small measure of "lightheartedness." Finally, a physically active life (brisk walks, jogging, or other aerobic activities) and a good night's sleep are certain to add extra years to your sojourn here on Earth.

Herbs to Grow and Use: Herbalists throughout the ages have always used heart-healthy herbs to protect and heal the cardiovascular system. The following herbs can be taken as teas (infusions or decoctions), tinctures, or in capsule form unless otherwise noted below.

- Cayenne, red clover, and rosemary in particular promote circulation, so include them regularly in baked dishes, sauces, or elixirs.

- Cayenne is a major ingredient in one of the greatest health tonics—salsa. Its spicy and heart-friendly ingredients (chiles, cilantro, garlic, onions, and tomatoes) and the savor it adds to foods help with digestion and are a boon to your palate and circulation alike.

- Garlic can be consumed regularly with meals to promote heart health.

- Hawthorn's traditional use is supported by modern science: It's the leading cardiovascular tonic that herbalists recommend.

- Hops reduces inflammation and promotes relaxation.

Heartburn

That burning sensation behind your breastbone, caused by a regurgitation of stomach acid, is often a result of stress and/or the consumption of spicy or irritating foods. This unpleasant malady can be accentuated by chronic gastritis or inflammation of your stomach, which may be associated with infection by the common bacteria *Helicobacter pylori*.

What Helps: Eating simply, especially if you include whole grains such as brown rice, quinoa, and millet, is very therapeutic. Rice gruel and barley water are perennial favorites for heartburn. Avoid fried foods, or coating any foods with oil, which delays digestion. Eat slowly and chew well.

Herbs to Grow and Use: The following herbs can be taken as teas (infusions or decoctions), tinctures, or in capsule form unless otherwise noted below.

- Chamomile, licorice, and marshmallow all have soothing properties and can be used as teas, ½ cup at a time, as needed throughout the day.

- Aloe helps, too. You can sip commercial aloe liquids or you can juice the inside of the leaf with a little celery or parsley to help counteract the acidic feel in your esophagus and throat.

Hormone Imbalances

Many hormones—estrogen, progesterone, cortisol, adrenaline, thyroid hormones, and others—are released by your body in response to input from your nervous system by way of your hypothalamus, as well as other stimuli. Because only minute amounts are required for a strong effect on the tissues and organs, hormones can dramatically affect mood and behavior. Since hormones are in delicate balance and interact with themselves and your nervous system, their regulation can be complex. Your liver also figures into the equation because it is the organ that breaks down hormones when your levels are too high, and it also happens to produce small amounts of estrogen, testosterone, and other hormones.

What Helps: A balanced diet containing moderate levels of protein, along with sufficient sleep, physical activity, and a positive attitude, will contribute to good hormonal balance. A regular yoga practice is helpful, as certain postures are intended to stimulate and balance specific glands. Stress is a complicated matter in our lives, since a small amount can be stimulating but too much will have a detrimental effect on hormone output. Our attitude toward stress is the key: It's not so much the actual stress, but how we handle it that counts.

Herbs to Grow and Use: The following herbs can be taken as teas (infusions or decoctions), tinctures, or in capsule form unless otherwise noted below.

- Red clover and vitex are two herbs we recommend to help balance sex hormones. Red clover has mild estrogen-balancing effects because of its phytoestrogens, such as genistein. Vitex increases progesterone levels while reducing and balancing other hormones that are associated with symptoms of premenstrual syndrome (PMS), such as mood swings, food cravings, and breast tenderness.

- Hops and lavender teas can both be used for relaxation and to destress, which is restorative to your hormonal system. You can also try ligustrum and rhodiola, since both are well known as support herbs during times of stress, especially benefitting mental work and energy.

- Licorice can support your adrenal function.

Hypertension

Hypertension, or high blood pressure, is a potentially serious chronic medical condition defined as a consistent systolic (heart contracting) reading of 140 or above and a diastolic (heart resting) reading of 90 or above. The two are expressed as a pair: 140/90. Hypertension is often a symptom of a wider range of problems in the body, especially chronic obesity, damage to and hardening of the blood vessels, and chronic stress, among others. Hypertension can greatly increase the possibility of early death due to strokes, heart attacks, and heart failure. It can arise when your blood vessels become chronically inflamed and eventually harden with deposits of lipids, proteins, calcium, and scar tissue.

What Helps: Following a heart-healthy program means strictly avoiding foods and drinks with added sugar; eating a low-sodium, high-potassium diet (one rich in green, leafy vegetables; moderating consumption of animal products like meat, dairy, and eggs; getting ample sleep and plenty of exercise; and reducing the impact of chronic stress. All of these practices can greatly reduce the incidence of and risks associated with hypertension. As with many natural and herbal programs, daily and regular use of herbs is essential for best results, which can be dramatic over time. Herbal adaptogens (which help our bodies deal with stress) are some of the most important herbs for hypertension and can help lessen the harmful impact of chronic stress. Herbs that nourish your liver are also key, since the liver regulates blood lipids and inflammatory pathways as part of your immune response.

Herbs to Grow and Use: The following herbs can be taken as teas (infusions or decoctions), tinctures, or in capsule form unless otherwise noted below.

- Garlic causes a modest reduction in blood pressure with regular use. Crush cloves first, then mix them into soups, chilis, salad dressings, and many other foods. A recommended dose is one to three cloves per day.

- Hawthorn and stevia, as research shows, can provide a mild but significant reduction of diastolic blood pressure when used regularly.

- Hops, applied in a steady maintenance dosage, can help promote a healthy inflammatory response.

- Turmeric—when added to food, taken as a decoction, or taken in capsules— is a superstar that can regulate inflammatory pathways with regular use.

- Artichoke is a refreshingly bitter liver and bile stimulant and can reduce cholesterol levels.

- Dandelion helps to maintain a healthy bile flow and support liver health. The bitter leaf can be added to salads, soups, and stir-fries.

Liver Health

Your liver carries out many vital functions, including detoxification, hormone production and regulation, digestive functions, and energy storage. Herbalists and other natural-care practitioners often think of your liver as a regulator and harmonizer of various aspects of your internal environment. As a result, liver imbalances are linked with such symptoms as emotional swings, irritability, and anger; headaches; red, itchy, dry eyes; and symptoms related to the menstrual cycle, such as PMS.

What Helps: Light caloric intake, regular bowel movements, healthy sleep, exercise, and a mostly vegetarian diet replete with whole grains, beans, vegetables, and fruits can all help your liver function at full capacity. This organ has to metabolize and detoxify all manner of pharmaceuticals and environmental chemicals (such as the PCBs we absorb from plastic), so eating organic foods and limiting your drug and alcohol use can give your liver a much-needed break.

Herbs to Grow and Use: The following herbs can be taken as teas (infusions or decoctions), tinctures, or in capsule form unless otherwise noted below.

- Burdock (the root is known as gobo) and turmeric are known to have strong liver-protective activity; use them regularly in cooking.

- Artichoke and Oregon grape will activate bile flow to keep digestion running smoothly.

- Ligustrum "moistens" and supports your liver and benefits your eyes.

- Take aloe, burdock, or red clover regularly to support your liver's detoxification efforts.

Memory Enhancement

Memory and recall are closely related to your cardiovascular health, in part because your brain needs a constant supply of energy and oxygen. When tiny blood vessels are even slightly narrowed, hardened, or blocked, a decline in mental ability will eventually follow. Mental decline, or dementia, can be one of the earliest signs of aging, and one of the most alarming.

What Helps: Good nutrition, exercise, and moderation in drug and alcohol use will help keep your blood flowing, protect your heart and blood vessels, and strengthen your memory and mental faculties. Using your mind by learning new things—even undertaking a major course of study every few years—will help keep your brain youthful.

Herbs to Grow and Use: The following herbs can be taken as teas (infusions or decoctions), tinctures, or in capsule form unless otherwise noted below.

- When used regularly, cayenne, garlic, hawthorn, red clover, and rosemary can all be used to help invigorate your circulation and protect your cardiovascular system.

- Gotu kola, hawthorn, red clover, and rosemary are especially effective at improving circulation.

- Rhodiola and gotu kola help improve memory and cognition.

Menopause and Maturity

The change of life for women (and men) comes in the late 40s or early 50s (although the process sometimes occurs later in men). This is the time when the focus in our lives turns from reproduction to other aspects of life. If we have taken good care of ourselves, our health and vitality can be good for another 30 years or more—time enough for a new career, volunteer work, relaxation, travel, education, renewing old acquaintances, and making new friends. It can also be a time of memories—of feeling wistful, nostalgic, proud, or wise.

Menopause and the changes it brings to our minds and bodies can also be difficult for some. Your feelings about aging can be accompanied by fatigue, hot flashes, changes in your sex drive, depression, and weight gain, among other symptoms.

What Helps: Exercising every day—stretching, walking, running—and a simple, whole-foods diet will always help to support your mood and bring a sense of physical well-being. You can also take a daily multivitamin supplement that contains whole-food extracts and other well-researched ingredients such as vitamin D, omega-3 fatty acids (including DHA and EPA), and anti-inflammatory herb extracts such as boswellia (*Boswellia serrata*), hops, and turmeric. This will help reduce chronic inflammation, which is the cause of many diseases (such as arthritis, heart disease, and diabetes). Watching your weight is important: You will feel better and live longer, since fat cells produce a number of inflammatory hormones that can promote chronic diseases.

A positive attitude and a good sense of humor work wonders. And since stress has a cumulative effect, make sure that you continue to use all the tools that are available to you: meditation, massage therapy, counseling, service work, spiritual affirmations, support groups, and therapeutic care of any kind. Cultivate friendships and community: It's never too late to make more friends, now that you have more time for giving and receiving friendship and love.

Herbs to Grow and Use: Menopause and the symptoms that sometimes accompany it can be effectively treated and even relieved through the use of natural remedies, including herbs. The following herbs can be taken as teas (infusions or decoctions), tinctures, or in capsule form unless otherwise noted below.

- Herbs for stress (adaptogens) can be used regularly for an extended time, especially if you find them helpful. These include ashwagandha, burdock, gotu kola, ligustrum, nettle, rhodiola, and tulsi basil (see "Stress Mitigation" on page 205).

- Herbs for relaxation and a good night's sleep include California poppy, chamomile, hawthorn, hops, lavender, lemon balm, and valerian.

- Hormone-balancing herbs include primarily those that contain a group of phytoestrogens (estrogenlike compounds) called isoflavones (such as genistein) from red clover, hops, and fennel. (Isoflavones are also found in soy extracts.) A progesterone-promoting herb that can also regulate other sex hormones (such as luteinizing hormone) is the well-known and widely recommended "women's herb," vitex.

- Herbs to balance your mood include St. John's wort and lavender.

- Herbs to support blood flow and reduce pelvic pain include angelica, ginger, and turmeric.

Mood Swings

Your mood is quite dependent on your overall physical health, your environment, and your attitude in life. You can cultivate and create happiness and emotional poise through practice and focus, and you can take care of your body and your immediate surroundings.

In traditional medicine throughout history, and across many cultures, strong emotions (depression, anxiety, anger, and fear) have been associated with the internal organs, and herbalists often treated the associated organ to help balance the emotion. These associations include:

- Digestive system and immune system: Worry and excessive mental work

- Heart (nervous and cardiovascular systems): Joy and mania

- Kidneys: Fear

- Liver: Irritability and anger

- Lungs: Grief

What Helps: A total program for emotional health and well-being can include regular sleeping hours, a healthy network of family and friends, meditation and/or spiritual practice, and as much exercise as possible, of various kinds. (Try gardening, dancing, biking, and frequent walking when other, more vigorous exercise is difficult or unavailable.) Healthy habits such as good nutrition and avoidance of refined sugar and excess caffeine can make a significant difference. Still, some mental and emotional swings are inherent in our busy and chaotic lives these days, and genetics do play a role. However, these influences are not "set in stone" and can be moderated through awareness and practice.

Many herbs and other dietary supplements can help us maintain a healthy emotional balance and stability. One B-vitamin capsule daily to ensure proper intake and a mineral blend in a whole-foods multivitamin can be very supportive, especially when your diet and nutrition are not perfect.

Herbs to Grow and Use: Herbalists often recommend paying attention to the health and balance of your liver, which is thought to be the main organ associated with moods and emotions. This is especially true when the emotions you feel are frequently irritation or anger, but also depression or anxiety. The following herbs can be taken as teas (infusions or decoctions), tinctures, or in capsule form unless otherwise noted below.

- Liver herbs to try are artichoke leaf, burdock, dandelion, Oregon grape, turmeric, wormwood, and yellow dock. With the exception of wormwood, these can be used freely on a regular basis to help maintain a healthy bile flow and liver balance.

- Herbs for maintaining emotional balance include California poppy, chamomile, gotu kola, hops, lavender, lemon balm, ligustrum, rhodiola, St. John's wort, valerian, and vitex.

Mucus Congestion

Mucus, or phlegm, is an important part of our natural defense against pathogens, trapping dust and other airborne particles that we might breathe in throughout the day and night. It can be copiously produced when you have an upper respiratory tract infection and your body is attempting to expel the viral pathogen.

Mucus can also be produced by your nasal sinuses during mild to severe respiratory allergies. It can become quite sticky and persistent as it makes its way into your throat, requiring frequent throat-clearing and coughing up of thick mucus discharge.

What Helps: Flushing your sinuses daily with a warm saline solution in an ear syringe or neti pot is widely recommended by physicians to remove wastes and allergens that can initiate allergic reactions and mucus discharge. Regular use of mucus-dissolving and decongesting herbs, as well as herbs that regulate the immune response and moderate inflammation, can be extremely effective at reducing unpleasant acute or chronic mucus discharge and congestion.

Herbs to Grow and Use: The following herbs can be taken as teas (infusions or decoctions), tinctures, or in capsule form unless otherwise noted below.

- Angelica tea, taken twice daily, can help calm an overactive immune response.

- Cayenne is hot, but it sure cuts the mucus in a hurry. Mix ¼ teaspoon in a little warm lemon water and drink it throughout the day to greatly speed the expectoration and elimination of mucus.

- Elder, goldenseal, and self-heal, used frequently throughout the day, can calm the allergic response.

- Mullein, peppermint, and rosemary are often effective at relieving congestion.

- Thyme and yerba mansa are effective antibacterial and antiviral herbs that help your body fight respiratory infections.

- Turmeric, used often in cooking (it's the main ingredient in curry) or in capsules or tinctures, is effective at reducing inflammation.

Muscle Strains and Sprains

Strains and sprains happen to all of us, but they are a lot more likely to happen when we don't stretch daily for at least 15 minutes (more preferably, up to 30 minutes) and keep our muscles, tendons, and ligaments strong with regular weight-bearing exercises and/or daily vigorous walking. Flopping down in the easy chair every day to watch the U.S. daily average of 6 hours of TV, then going on a "kick" at the gym or attempting to go back to the way we used to do the Warrior 1 pose at yoga class is a classic way to sustain an injury.

What Helps: The best thing you can do is to undertake daily stretching, yoga, walking, dancing, gardening, or any other physical activity that involves moving and stretching your body in various ways—making sure that you warm up if the activity is vigorous. Our bodies are meant to move, and the more, the better (short of obsession, of course). And you can try hydrotherapy (alternating hot and cold water on your body) to prevent strains and sprains. It's an ancient, traditional way to keep blood circulating to your muscles and joints. We recommend finishing a hot shower with a cool one: Just reach up and turn down the hot water at the end so that you expose your whole body to the coolness. It's a wonderful feeling that is refreshing and restoring, closing your pores and improving skin health. Work up to a completely cold shower for extra circulatory benefits. It will make you tingle all over, especially if you live in the northern climes.

Herbs to Grow and Use: The following herbs can be taken as teas (infusions or decoctions), tinctures, or in capsule form unless otherwise noted below. Herbs to improve circulation and promote healing also work well when applied as compresses or added to baths.

- Either alone or combined, strong ginger and rosemary tea can speed healing and provide fast relief for stiff, sore muscles when applied as a compress or added to a bath.

- Turmeric is a great herb for reducing inflammation and pain when taken orally for a few weeks at a time.

Nausea

Nausea is a symptom that can be caused by many things: certain diseases, eating spoiled food, overeating, intestinal gas buildup, morning sickness (common during early pregnancy), motion sickness (such as from riding in the back seat of a car or in a boat over choppy waves), and even stressful and highly emotional situations. As we all know, nausea is an unpleasant feeling and really gets our attention. When nausea continues for more than a day or two, consult your physician or health-care provider.

What Helps: For nausea associated with overeating, eating too quickly, or poor food combinations, pressing on and massaging your abdominal area will sometimes rapidly relieve the symptom.

A warm ginger compress on your stomach is often effective, as are several acupressure points. (One is located in the webbing between your thumb and first finger, and another is located on your wrist. You can buy pressure bracelets that activate the points to prevent motion sickness.)

Herbs to Grow and Use: Fortunately, a few herbs have been shown to really help reduce nausea quickly. The following herbs can be taken as teas (infusions or decoctions), tinctures, or in capsule form unless otherwise noted below.

- For nausea that occurs along with a stomach flu or other infection, sip echinacea tea throughout the day.

- Ginger is the most proven herb for reducing nausea and is widely recommended by herbalists. If you don't feel relief within 15 to 30 minutes of taking ginger, increase the frequency or size of your dosage.

- Other herbs that have been shown to help you calm down and relieve digestive distress include chamomile (a strong cup of tea every hour or two), fennel or peppermint (in tea, tablet, or candy form, especially when symptoms are due to gas buildup), lavender (tea, aromatherapy or bath), and wormwood. (See page 98 for wormwood's dosage guidance.)

Nerve Pain (*Neuralgia*)

Chronic nerve pain can be associated with a number of chronic ailments, such as diabetes, herpes, chronic fatigue syndrome, and fibromyalgia. Acute nerve pain often follows an injury, sometimes goes along with caffeine withdrawal, may come after overly ambitious physical activity you are not used to (such as running a marathon without adequate preparation), or be present during an infection such as a bad flu.

What Helps: Massage, gentle stretching, and hydrotherapy. (See "Muscle Strains and Sprains" on page 198.) Try bathing or showering in warm or hot water followed by a cool or cold shower at a ratio of 4:1 minutes, several times daily. You can also adapt this to a sauna or locally to a compress.

Herbs to Grow and Use: The following herbs can be taken as teas (infusions or decoctions), tinctures, or in capsule form unless otherwise noted below.

- For nearly 2,000 years, St. John's wort, internally and externally, has been and remains certainly one of the most widely recommended remedies to help relieve nerve pain. Apply the oil liberally to affected areas at least two or three times daily. Take tinctures, capsules, or tablets two or three times a day. (See page 89 for information on potential drug and herb interactions.)

- Other herbs that help reduce nerve pain when used regularly are anti-inflammatory herbs such as ginger, rosemary, and turmeric. These work well as compresses or in baths.

Nervousness

Feelings of nervousness, edginess, agitation, and anxiety are experienced— probably frequently—by people every- where in this modern age (and likely since the Stone Age). These feelings are a natural response to danger, either perceived or real. They alert us to the potential for harm if we don't pay attention and don't act. Nervousness, edginess, and even anxiety make sense when a dangerous animal is chasing us, but what about when we are hurtling down the freeway at 70 miles per hour in a small metal box with a lot of other, much bigger boxes, coming straight for us? Freeway driving may be routine, but our nervous system and fight-or-flight mechanisms are still highly aroused by it.

Besides physical danger, our nervous and hormonal systems are frequently alerted throughout the day and even the night (if you have an apartment in a big city) by background noise, the incessant stimulation of computers, the e-mail barrage, adrenaline-pumping movies and media, the consumption of stimulating beverages, and, no doubt, through intense or uncomfortable personal interactions and conflicts.

What Helps: Taking the time to focus and calm down really helps. Usually this involves removing yourself from overstimulating situations, just as you would settle a child by reading a peaceful and heartwarming story before bedtime. Take the time to withdraw, and pay attention to the signals that let you know you've had too much stimulation. Try a regular practice of taking a calming stroll with no goal in mind except to enjoy.

You'll find many other healthy suggestions in the realm of self-help books, and you might discover great restorative power in peaceful ocean soundscapes or relaxing music. Stress-related support groups are widely available and highly valuable. Yoga, tai chi, dancing, running clubs, bird-watching groups, native plant societies, meditation groups, and spiritual practices are all wonderful healing islands, as well.

Herbs to Grow and Use: Not surprisingly, many herbs can relieve stress and calm your nervous system, engendering a sense of peace and promoting refreshing sleep. They can be taken as teas (infusions or decoctions), tinctures, or in capsule form unless otherwise noted below.

- California poppy contains nonnarcotic alkaloids that help promote calm and good sleep.

- Catnip, chamomile, lemon balm, lemon verbena, and skullcap are all very mild herbs for calming that are safe for kids and can be used in baths.

- Gotu kola is an excellent tonic herb for the nervous system.

- Hawthorn is a great heart and digestive herb that has mild calming effects, especially when used regularly.

- Hops promotes good sleep and calm. Nonalcoholic "hoppy" beers such as Clausthaler contain high levels of the herb.

- Lavender is widely used in inhalants and in baths to create a sense of relaxation.

- Rhodiola is an excellent adaptogen and nerve and brain tonic.

- St. John's wort is often recommended to help prevent and reduce the symptoms of depression and anxiety, especially when it's used regularly and continuously. Be aware of cautions regarding drug interactions (see page 89).

- Valerian is probably the most widely recommended calming and sleep-promoting herb. Freshly harvested roots and rhizomes have stronger and more calming activity than the dried herb.

Pain, General

Pain is nature's wake-up call. If we ignore minor pain, it may eventually get worse. Spending most of our time sitting in front of a computer or TV can result in lower back pain. However, injuries and accidents can also lead to pain, and chronic internal diseases such as heart disease, diabetes, and cancer send pain signals as well. According to traditional systems of healing, such as traditional Chinese medicine, pain is the result of stagnation of blood and vital energy.

What Helps: The recommended treatment for pain in traditional Chinese medicine is to "move the blood and vital energy." In Western terms, this means bringing more healing nutrients and beneficial immune cells to the area and stimulating the nerves to reduce pain signals. You can often accomplish this through massage, acupuncture, stretching, exercise, and herbs.

Herbs to Grow and Use: The following herbs can be taken as teas (infusions or decoctions), tinctures, or in capsule form unless otherwise noted below.

- Ginger is probably the best example of an herb that gets the energy and blood moving. You can capture its warming nature by making a strong tea to use in compresses and baths and by combining it with rosemary for added effect.

- The most famous pain-relieving herb is the opium poppy (*Papaver somnifera*). It can be argued that no man-made drug is as effective as this ancient, naturally occurring plant. Though its use is old, growing it is illegal throughout the United States and other parts of the world. However, you can also use another herb in the poppy family, California poppy, to gently reduce pain, especially from cramps.

- For the pain of injuries, apply cayenne cream, along with other herbal essential oils, especially camphor, clove (*Syzygium aromaticum*), rosemary, and wintergreen (*Gaultheria shallon*). (Caution—don't use wintergreen internally.)

- St. John's wort oil, applied liberally several times daily, is an excellent remedy for nerve pain and other injuries.

- For any pain, use turmeric and/or ginger to gently reduce inflammation over a few days to a few weeks.

Premenstrual Syndrome (PMS)

Premenstrual syndrome is a collection of symptoms including depression, irritability, food cravings, water retention, breast tenderness, acne, and constipation that can occur prior to the onset of menses during a woman's monthly cycle. During menstruation, some women experience cramping and some of the same symptoms mentioned above due to rapid changes in levels of estrogen, progesterone, and other hormones.

What Helps: Taking good care of yourself is crucial when PMS hits. Be restful and pamper yourself if you can, take warm herbal baths and apply warm compresses, and get a loving massage from a partner or friend. (Use an herbal oil such as St. John's wort oil.) Take a multivitamin and other nutritional supplements, such as magnesium, calcium, and essential fatty acids. Add additional dark, leafy greens and lean protein, such as fish, to your diet (they contain high levels of magnesium and B vitamins) to help with cramping and mood swings.

Herbs to Grow and Use: Herbalists will tend to recommend herbal hormone regulators and "blood-regulating" herbs (those that enhance circulation and fortify the blood), and they often associate PMS with a congested liver condition. Adaptogenic herbs, calming herbs, pain-relieving herbs, and herbal sleep aids can all help ease the symptoms. The following herbs can be taken as teas (infusions or decoctions), tinctures, or in capsule form unless otherwise noted below.

- Herbs that assist liver function include artichoke and burdock.

- Herbs to relieve cramping include California poppy, chamomile, lavender, valerian, vitex, and yarrow.

- We recommend ashwagandha, gotu kola, rhodiola, and tulsi basil as adaptogens to help with hormonal balance and energy and to regulate mood.

- St. John's wort can be helpful for both anxiety and depression, and valerian is one of the best sleep herbs.

- Vitex has been known for centuries to be an important female hormone regulator and is widely taken for relieving the symptoms of PMS.

Skin Ailments

Skin ailments, such as rashes, acne, boils, styes, psoriasis, and eczema are difficult to diagnose and can occur on any part of your body. Keeping your body's channels of elimination open allows your liver to excrete bile and your gut to dispose of urine and waste efficiently, which is essential to beautiful, clear skin.

Rashes and eczema can be a visible outer response to an allergic reaction. Allergies to foods such as soy, wheat, dairy, and eggs are common. We also react to chemicals in the environment, and many of them—pesticides, herbicides, and ingredients in body-care and cleaning products, for example—are invisible to the eye. Because they are completely foreign to your immune system, it tries to rid your body of them, which can create a strong inflammatory response that shows up on your skin.

Acne and boils, which are infections occurring inside your skin, can sometimes be traced to skin or gut imbalances and impaired elimination.

What Helps: Buying and growing organic foods and using natural body-care products, laundry soap, and dish-washing detergents is extremely important for maintaining good skin health. And remember to use caution when choosing a body soap. Soap can wash away natural fatty acids that help keep your skin's eco-system in balance. Believe it or not, many bacteria live *inside* your skin, not on the surface, so the use of a probiotic supplement can help. An imbalance in your skin's microflora is closely associated with a strong imbalance in your gut's microflora. Following a healthy, simple diet that includes lots of fresh fruits and veggies is a key step to good skin health. A daily intake of "prebiotics," which are foods high in soluble fiber, such as beans or whole oats, can encourage good overall skin health. We recommend keeping a fiber "report card" for yourself. Your body's short-term and long-term health depend on a high intake of fiber every day.

Herbs to Grow and Use: Good digestion is essential for avoiding skin ailments and maintaining a high level of skin health. Many of the herbs mentioned in the "Digestive Problems" and "Liver Health" sections (see pages 186 and 194) are recommended by herbalists for relieving and avoiding rashes, acne, boils, and other inflammatory skin conditions. The following herbs can be taken as teas (infusions or decoctions), tinctures, or in capsule form unless otherwise noted below.

- Herbs to activate the bile and promote detoxification include aloe, artichoke, burdock, Oregon grape, red clover, and turmeric.

- Herbs to calm your immune response and directly benefit your skin include angelica, elder, honeysuckle, nettle, and red clover.

Sleep Problems

How important is restful and adequate sleep to your overall health? A well-publicized study from Carnegie Mellon in 2009 showed that volunteers who were exposed to a cold virus and had less than 7 hours of sleep per night for the 2 weeks prior to the study had three times the likelihood of coming down with cold symptoms than those who got more than 8 hours per night. And researchers from the Mayo Clinic found that people who got less sleep than the recommended 8 hours received less protection from the flu vaccine.

It's remarkable that although we might know the importance of sleep, we still rarely give ourselves enough of it. The National Sleep Foundation has reported that the U.S. average is about 6.7 hours a night, and the overall trend is downward. Besides that decline, it is noteworthy that the quality of our sleep is not getting any better, either. Noise and light pollution affects many of us these days, even during the night. Pharmaceutical and recreational drug and alcohol use can also strongly decrease delta (deep) and REM (dreaming) sleep, which are both vital to receiving the healing and restorative benefits of sleep.

What Helps: If you need help with noise and light pollution, wear earplugs and draw the blinds or curtains. Stretch, relax, stop working, and avoid heavy foods and stimulating drinks in the evening. A relaxing walk before bedtime can help clear your mind and settle your emotions. Vigorous exercise or physical work earlier in the day benefits us in many ways, including by improving our sleep. While one glass of wine or one beer around dinnertime can help us relax and is not likely to affect our sleep quality significantly, heavy drinking and recreational drugs, especially when used late in the evening, can.

Herbs to Grow and Use: Herbs have a long history of use for promoting good sleep. The following herbs can be taken as teas (infusions or decoctions), tinctures, or in capsule form unless otherwise noted below.

- No herb is as notable a sleep aid as valerian. In 2011, researchers from Tehran University conducted a well-designed blinded study including 100 postmenopausal women with insomnia. They found that 30 percent of the women in the valerian group reported better sleep quality, including falling asleep faster and waking up less at night. Only 4 percent of the women in the placebo group reported improved sleep. Valerian preparations vary widely in their quality and effects; see page 94 for more information.

- Other herbs recommended by herbalists for improving sleep include California poppy, chamomile, hops, and lavender.

- If you are helping young children to relax and sleep, try gentle herbs such as California poppy, catnip, and lemon balm.

Sore Throat

A really sore throat is not fun. Have you ever had one bad enough that you had to get up your courage to even swallow? A sore throat is a symptom that is sometimes present in the first stages of a respiratory tract infection like a cold or flu, and it often reduces in severity after a few days.

What Helps: Gargling with a mild salt solution can reduce swelling and discomfort and can be very helpful. Gargle frequently throughout the day, as often as every 30 to 60 minutes. Place a humidifier in the room if you live in a place where the air is dry, perhaps adding a calming essential oil like lavender to the water. Drink warm or cool liquids, depending on your preference, to ensure ample hydration, especially when you have a fever.

Herbs to Grow and Use: Soothing and healing plant essences bring pain relief and other side benefits. The following herbs can be taken as teas (infusions or decoctions), tinctures, or in capsule form unless otherwise noted below.

- The top herb to treat a sore throat is garden sage. We often go out to the garden and pick a few tender leaves to chew on, swallowing the juice. Drinking the tea throughout the day works well, too.

- Frequently use herbs that prevent bacterial growth and reduce soreness: anise hyssop, chamomile, lavender, red clover, rosemary, St. John's wort, and thyme.

- Soothing herbs with a high mucilage content or anti-inflammatory properties for coating and soothing include comfrey, licorice, and marshmallow.

Stress Mitigation

Many of us are likely to agree that stress can affect our immune response, and early 1993 research at Carnegie Mellon University confirms this. Among 394 healthy volunteers, those under the highest amount of stress had consistently more cold symptoms when they were exposed to the virus. Many kinds of stress are present today: irritating sounds or noises, environmental pollution, emotional and interpersonal conflicts, worry about work or the state of the world, overstimulation from media, and increasing responsibilities. However, it's not so much the actual stress that adversely affects our health, but rather how we respond to and deal with it.

What Helps: Can you let stress roll off your back like water off a duck, or do you take it to heart and make it personal? The choice is often yours, but it takes a daily practice of meditation, yoga, or other discipline, as well as frequent exercise, to help with this lifetime project. Along with the exercise, sleep is an important shield against the harmful effects of stress. Ironically, your sleep is often adversely affected under stress, which can lead to a vicious circle of stress leading to poor sleep, which then leads to more stress. And if we aren't able to develop positive habits and techniques to relieve and release stress, we often turn to drugs and alcohol, which can add their own harmful stresses to our lives.

Our advice echoes that of many holistic practitioners today that have recommended ways to relieve the harmful effects of stress. The fact that many of these were once considered "alternative therapies" but are now household words points to their effectiveness if adopted: daily yoga, meditation or a spiritual practice, exercise, massage or other holistic therapeutics, as well as positive visualization. Pets, professional counseling, support groups, and a healthy circle of close friends and family will further reduce the effect stress has on you.

Herbs to Grow and Use: Herbs to relieve the harmful effects of stress and regulate and normalize all of the body systems, especially the hormonal, nervous, and immune systems, are called adaptogens. A number of adaptogens have been identified and studied, and entire books have been written on their benefits. The following herbs can be taken as teas (infusions or decoctions), tinctures, or in capsule form unless otherwise noted below.

- The best-studied adaptogens, from a scientific perspective, include eleuthero or Siberian ginseng (*Eleutherococcus senticosis*), rhodiola, tulsi basil, reishi (*Ganoderma lucidum*), and American ginseng (*Panax quinquefolium*).

- Ligustrum is a special adaptogen that can help restore balance to all of your body systems.

- Astragalus acts as an adaptogen-like strengthening tonic for your immune system.

- Ashwagandha helps counteract stress and promotes relaxation.

- Burdock (sometimes known as gobo) and nettle act as strengthening tonics and help to eliminate the buildup of waste products produced by a stressed system.

- Gotu kola promotes clear thinking and is considered a brain and nervous system tonic when used regularly.

- Hawthorn is a tonic for the heart and cardiovascular system, which are taxed during periods of heavy stress.

- Rhodiola helps promote balance and vitality, especially for the nervous system and mental faculties.

Ulcers

An ulcer is an opening in a bodily membrane that can be inflamed and painful, disrupting the proper function of the tissue. An ulcer can appear on the surface of your skin as a result of an infectious disease, cancer, a burn, or an injury. When you hear the word "ulcer," you might think of a *gastric* ulcer, which is an erosion of the membrane inside the stomach or adjoining duodenum (the upper portion of the small intestine). In recent years, stomach ulcers have been associated with an overgrowth of the bacteria *Helicobacter pylori*. A high percentage of the population has *H. pylori* in their stomachs, but ulcers only occur in some people that carry the bacteria. Antiulcer medications are commonly sold over the counter and have been among the top sellers for many years—a testament to the universal occurrence of this ailment.

What Helps: For some of us, the stomach is long-suffering. It must endure everything that goes into our mouths—pepperoni pizza, barbecued ribs, deep-fried onion rings, and cola drinks laced with tooth- and stomach-eroding acids. A 2010 study at the McGill Faculty of Dentistry in Montreal found that some soft drinks have a pH of 5.5, which is strongly acidic. Scanning electron microscopic analysis of tooth surfaces after volunteers gargled with various soft drinks clearly showed erosion of the enamel.

To help prevent gastric ulcers from occurring in the first place, follow a high-fiber diet including lots of veggies, fruits, whole grains, and beans. Strictly avoid soft drinks of all kinds, substituting water or sparkling water mixed with a little unsweetened fruit juice, which has a higher pH and lower potential for erosion of your teeth and mucous membranes.

Stress is strongly associated with the formation of ulcers (see "Stress Mitigation" on page 205).

Herbs to Grow and Use: Herbs to help prevent and reduce the symptoms of a gastric ulcer include soothing mucilaginous herbs, inflammation-reducing herbs, antibacterial herbs that contain the constituent berberine (which inhibits *H. pylori* growth), and antistress herbs (known as adaptogens). You can take the following herbs in tea (either infusions or decoctions) or capsule form.

- Aloe, comfrey, and marshmallow can be taken frequently throughout the day when symptoms flare up. For prevention, a cup twice daily in combination with an anti-inflammatory herb such as licorice or St. John's wort will work well.

- Anti-inflammatory herbs include chamomile, licorice, and yarrow. Three others bear special mention: gotu kola, Oregon grape, and St. John's wort, which are traditional herbs for reducing inflammation in the gastrointestinal tract and which can also reduce *H. pylori* levels and promote healing. Take gotu kola as a fresh juice, if you can (see page 42). You can freeze any that is left over at the end of the growing season. Take capsules or the extract if these are the only forms available; they will work well, too. St. John's wort is used in Europe in the form of an oil (see page 168). You can take 1 teaspoon at a time, one or two times daily, as well as use the tea and capsules. Exercise caution with St. John's wort preparations if you are taking pharmaceuticals, and follow the cautions in this herb's profile on page 89.

- Antibacterial herbs like aloe gel and Oregon grape can be added to the other herbs recommended above in teas or taken in capsule form.

- Antistress or adaptogenic herbs such as gotu kola, ligustrum, rhodiola and tulsi basil are helpful when treating an ulcer caused by stress.

Urinary Tract Infections and Frequent Urination

Urinary tract infections (UTIs) are quite common, especially in women. In one 2002 review from the University of Michigan School of Public Health, the authors reported that UTIs were responsible for nearly 7 million doctor visits and 1 million emergency room visits that year. The researchers emphasized that these figures were likely to be very low because physicians are not required to report UTIs in the United States. Nearly one in three women have at least one UTI requiring antibiotics by the age of 24, and nearly half will have a UTI sometime in her lifetime.

Symptoms of a UTI can include burning and painful urination and increased frequency or urge to urinate, even to the point that it disturbs your sleep at night. Up to 80 percent of UTIs are thought to be caused by the common gut bacteria *E. coli*, which explains why women are more likely to experience UTIs than men: The perineum (the short distance between the anus and the opening of the labia) is often colonized with *E. coli*, which can easily migrate up to the opening of the short urethra and then

into the bladder. A 2012 study at the University of Florida showed that, among young college women experiencing their first UTI, alcohol and coffee consumption, recent sexual activity, and number of partners were all closely correlated factors.

What Helps: You can drink unsweetened cranberry juice twice daily to help prevent bacteria from attaching to the bladder wall and causing an infection. A 2004 review of studies of the association of food intake with the incidence of UTIs showed that a diet high in berries, fruit juices, and fermented milk products like kefir or yogurt can help to reduce the incidence and recurrence of infections in women. Probiotic products containing *Lactobacillus* organisms are effective at preventing UTIs and reducing the symptoms and recurrences of UTIs by helping to maintain healthy microflora in the gut and in the vaginal area, according to 2011 research from Barkatullah University in India. The researchers point out that maintaining a slightly acidic environment in the genital area can help discourage *E. coli* colonization and reduce infections. A probiotic douche once a month, or daily during an active infection, can help maintain this environment if you are prone to UTIs.

Herbs to Grow and Use: Herbalists have recommended herbal formulas to reduce the incidence of UTIs for at least 400 years. These helpful herbs fall into several categories and can all be taken as teas (either infusions or decoctions), tinctures, and in capsule form.

- Immune boosters to support your body's process to fight and prevent infections: andrographis, echinacea, garlic, thyme, tulsi basil, and yerba mansa.

- Herbal diuretics to flush and help cleanse the urinary tract: dandelion, hops, love-in-a-mist, nettle, and yarrow.

- Antibacterial herbs: garlic, hops, lavender, love-in-a-mist, oregano, Oregon grape, rosemary, sage, thyme, yarrow, and lemon verbena.

- Anti-inflammatory herbs: aloe gel, chamomile, gotu kola, lemon balm, licorice, marshmallow, Oregon grape, St. John's wort, turmeric, and yarrow.

- Soothing mucilaginous herbs: comfrey, marshmallow, mullein, nettle, and plantain.

USING HERBS IN PREPARATIONS

HERB	PRIMARY USES	DOSE	SAFE IN PREGNANCY?	
Aloe *Aloe vera*	Heals skin trauma (external use); soothes and heals stomach and intestines (internal use).	Apply gel as needed to skin (external use); drink 4 to 6 ounces of juice 2 or 3 times daily (internal use).	Do not use without the advice of an expert or experienced herbalist	
Andrographis *Andrographis paniculata*	Prevents and shortens duration of colds, flu, and infections.	Take 1 or 2 capsules or tablets 3 times daily.	Use caution	
Angelica *Angelica archangelica*	Aids digestion; improves circulation; acts as a bitter tonic.	Take 1 dropperful of tincture before meals.	Not recommended	
Anise hyssop *Agastache foeniculum*	Aids digestion; eases colds and flu.	Drink 1 cup infusion 2 or 3 times daily.	Considered safe	
Artichoke *Cynara scolymus*	Aids digestion through its bitter action; balances cholesterol.	Take 1 to 2 droppersful of tincture or 2 capsules or tablets, 2 or 3 times daily.	Considered safe	
Ashwagandha *Withania somnifera*	Balances all body systems; increases energy; relieves arthritis; reduces anxiety.	Drink 1 cup decoction or take 2 or 3 capsules or tablets, twice daily.	Do not use without the advice of an expert or experienced herbalist	
Astragalus *Astragalus membranaceus*	Boosts energy and immune response.	Drink 1 cup decoction or take 1 or 2 capsules or tablets, 2 or 3 times daily.	Considered safe	
Basil and Tulsi *Ocimum basilicum* and *O. tenuiflorum*, syn. *O. sanctum*	Benefits nervous system and digestion.	Drink 1 cup infusion 2 or 3 times daily; use in cooking.	Use caution, except in cooking	
Burdock *Arctium lappa*	Improves energy; cleanses body systems; benefits liver.	Drink 1 cup decoction 2 or 3 times daily; use in cooking.	Considered safe	
Calendula *Calendula officinalis*	Treats skin conditions (external use).	Apply salve or cream as needed to skin.	Considered safe for external use	
California poppy *Eschscholzia californica*	Calms; promotes sleep.	Take 1 to 2 droppersful tincture or 1 or 2 capsules or tablets, 2 or 3 times daily.	No safety concerns known	
Catnip *Nepeta cataria*	Lowers fever; calms children.	Drink $\frac{1}{2}$ to 1 cup infusion several times daily.	Use caution	
Cayenne *Capsicum annuum*	Relieves pain (external use); clears mucus congestion and benefits circulation (internal use).	Apply as needed (external use); drink $\frac{1}{4}$ teaspoon powdered herb in hot water or take 2 capsules, 2 or 3 times daily (internal use).	No safety concerns for external use; moderate internal use considered safe	
Chamomile, German and Roman *Matricaria recutita* and *Chamaemelum nobile*, syn. *Anthemis nobilis*	Calms digestion (for the whole family).	Drink 2 to 4 cups infusion daily.	No safety concerns	

| | | | | CAN BE USED IN | | | | |
Infusions	Decoctions	Dried Teas	Bath Teas	Syrups	Tinctures	Oils	Compresses	Creams, Lotions, and Salves
		Yes		Yes				Yes
Yes		Yes		Yes	Yes			
	Yes	Yes		Yes	Yes			
Yes			Yes	Yes	Yes			
Yes		Yes		Yes	Yes			
	Yes	Yes			Yes			
	Yes	Yes						
Yes				Yes	Yes	Yes	Yes	Yes
	Yes	Yes			Yes			
			Yes			Yes	Yes	Yes
	Yes	Yes		Yes	Yes			
Yes			Yes	Yes				
				Yes	Yes	Yes	Yes	Yes
Yes			Yes	Yes	Yes	Yes	Yes	Yes

(continued)

USING HERBS IN PREPARATIONS (continued)

HERB	PRIMARY USES	DOSE	SAFE IN PREGNANCY?	
Comfrey *Symphytum officinalis*	Promotes healing of wounds, burns, and other skin trauma; relieves aches and pains (external use).	Apply liberally to affected areas, avoiding open wounds.	No safety concerns for external use on unbroken skin	
Echinacea *Echinacea purpurea, E. angustifolia*	Stimulates immune system to prevent and treat colds, flu, and infections.	Drink 2 to 4 cups infusion daily, or take 2 to 4 capsules or tablets or 2 to 4 droppersful tincture, every 2 to 3 hours.	Considered safe	
Elder *Sambucus nigra, ssp. canadensis/caerulea, syn. S. nigra, S. canadensis, S. mexicana*	Reduces fevers (flower); treats flu and skin ailments (berry).	Drink 2 to 4 cups infusion daily, or take 1 teaspoon berry syrup 3 times daily.	Considered safe	
Fennel *Foeniculum vulgare*	Improves digestion and relieves gas.	Drink 1 cup infusion after meals as needed.	Use caution	
Garlic *Allium sativum*	Benefits cardiovascular system; helps fight sinus and throat infections; treats cancer.	Eat 1 clove crushed in food 2 or 3 times daily, or take $\frac{1}{4}$ teaspoon syrup as needed.	Considered safe	
Gotu kola *Centella asiatica, syn. Hydrocotyle asiatica*	Improves memory (traditional use); calms; benefits cardiovascular system and skin conditions.	Drink 1 to 4 ounces juice or 2 to 3 cups infusion daily, or take 2 or 3 capsules or tablets 1 to 4 times daily (internal use); apply cream as needed (external use).	Considered safe	
Hawthorn *Crataegus laevigata, C. oxycantha, and C. pinnatifida*	Protects the heart and promotes cardiovascular health.	Drink 1 to 2 cups infusion daily or take 2 or 3 capsules or tablets 2 times daily.	Considered safe	
Honeysuckle *Lonicera japonica*	Treats flu, fevers, and other respiratory infections; acts as an antiviral.	Drink 1 cup infusion 2 or 3 times daily.	Considered safe	
Hops *Humulus lupulus*	Calms and promotes sleep; aids digestion.	Drink $\frac{1}{2}$ to 1 cup infusion or take 2 droppersful tincture, 2 times daily.	Considered safe	
Lavender *Lavandula angustifolia*	Calms and soothes the body, mind and spirit (internal and external use).	Drink 1 cup infusion 2 or 3 times daily (internal use); apply as needed (aromatherapy and external use).	Considered safe	
Lemon balm *Melissa officinalis*	Soothes herpes sores (external use); settles and relaxes the stomach and nerves (internal use).	Apply topically twice daily (external use); drink 1 cup infusion as desired (internal use).	Considered safe	
Lemon verbena *Aloysia citriodora, syn. A. triphylla*	Aids digestion; calms and promotes sleep.	Drink 1 cup infusion 2 or 3 times daily and before bed.	No safety concerns known	

			CAN BE USED IN					
Infusions	Decoctions	Dried Teas	Bath Teas	Syrups	Tinctures	Oils	Compresses	Creams, Lotions, and Salves
Yes (leaf)	Yes (root)						Yes	Yes
	Yes	Yes		Yes	Yes		Yes	Yes
Yes				Yes	Yes			Yes
Yes				Yes	Yes			
				Yes	Yes	Yes		
Yes		Yes	Yes	Yes	Yes		Yes	Yes
	Yes	Yes		Yes	Yes			
Yes		Yes	Yes	Yes	Yes			
Yes				Yes	Yes			
Yes			Yes	Yes	Yes	Yes	Yes	Yes
Yes		Yes	Yes	Yes	Yes			Yes
Yes			Yes	Yes	Yes	Yes		Yes

(continued)

HERB	PRIMARY USES	DOSE	SAFE IN PREGNANCY?	
Licorice *Glycyrrhiza glabra,* *G. uralensis*	Dissolves mucus; reduces inflammation and irritation of digestive and respiratory tracts; masks taste of bitter herbs.	Drink ½ cup decoction twice daily, alone or blended with other herbs.	Considered safe when used moderately (less than ¼ ounce dried herb per day)	
Ligustrum *Ligustrum lucidum*	Strengthens the immune system and liver function; balances the hormonal system; counteracts stress and fatigue.	Drink 1 cup infusion or take 1 to 2 droppersful tincture 2 or 3 times daily; also available in combination products as capsules or tablets.	No safety concerns known	
Love-in-a-mist *Nigella damascena*	Benefits digestive and respiratory tracts; relieves gas; promotes energy.	Drink 1 cup infusion twice daily; use in cooking.	No safety concerns known	
Marshmallow *Althaea officinalis*	Soothes digestive, respiratory, and urinary tracts.	Drink 2 to 3 cups infusion daily.	Considered safe	
Mullein *Verbascum* spp.	Soothes ears (flower oil); relieves mucus congestion and reduces irritation of the respiratory tract (leaf infusion).	Place 2 or 3 drops oil in the ear as needed and before bed; drink 1 cup leaf infusion 2 or 3 times daily.	Considered safe	
Nettle *Urtica dioica, U.* spp.	Benefits urinary tract; reduces allergy symptoms; acts as a strengthening mineral tonic.	Drink 2 to 3 cups infusion daily as needed; steam leaves in culinary dishes.	Considered safe	
Oregano *Origanum vulgare*	Treats upper respiratory tract infections; relieves gas.	Drink 2 to 3 cups strong infusion as needed; use in cooking.	Infusion and culinary use considered safe; avoid oil	
Oregon grape *Mahonia aquifolium*	Relieves acne and other skin problems; treats infections of all kinds.	Drink 1 to 2 cups decoction daily combined with other herbs (for bitterness).	Not recommended	
Peppermint and Spearmint *Mentha x piperita* and *M. spicata*	Relieves gas and digestive and respiratory tract discomfort.	Drink ½ to 1 cup infusion as needed.	Considered safe	
Red clover *Trifolium pratense*	Treats menopausal symptoms; acts as an expectorant and blood purifier; taken in many herbal cleansing programs.	Drink 1 cup infusion 2 or 3 times daily, or take 1 or 2 capsules or tablets 2 or 3 times daily.	Do not use without the advice of an expert or experienced herbalist	
Rhodiola *Rhodiola rosea*	Counteracts stress and fatigue; promotes vitality and good mental and immune function.	Take 1 to 2 droppersful tincture or 1 or 2 capsules or tablets, twice daily.	Do not use without the advice of an expert or experienced herbalist	
Rosemary *Rosmarinus officinalis*	Acts as an energizing antioxidant; benefits memory.	Drink 1 to 2 cups infusion, or take 1 to 2 droppersful tincture daily; use in baths.	Not recommended internally, especially the essential oil	
Sage *Salvia officinalis*	Reduces discomfort of sore throat; acts as an antibacterial for upper respiratory tract infections.	Sip 1 to 2 cups infusion daily, as needed.	Not recommended	

| | CAN BE USED IN | | | | | | | |
Infusions	Decoctions	Dried Teas	Bath Teas	Syrups	Tinctures	Oils	Compresses	Creams, Lotions, and Salves
	Yes	Yes		Yes	Yes			
	Yes	Yes		Yes	Yes			
Yes				Yes	Yes			
	Yes	Yes		Yes	Yes			Yes
Yes				Yes	Yes	Yes	Yes	
Yes		Yes	Yes					
Yes						Yes	Yes	
	Yes	Yes			Yes		Yes	Yes
Yes			Yes	Yes		Yes	Yes	Yes
Yes		Yes		Yes	Yes			Yes
		Yes			Yes			
Yes			Yes	Yes	Yes	Yes	Yes	Yes
Yes								

(continued)

HERB	PRIMARY USES	DOSE	SAFE IN PREGNANCY?	
Self-heal, heal all *Prunella vulgaris*	Acts as an antiviral for colds and flu; cleanses the liver; benefits the skin.	Drink 2 to 3 cups infusion daily, or take 2 to 3 droppersful tincture twice daily.	No safety concerns known	
Skullcap *Scutellaria lateriflora*	Reduces nervousness, anxiety, and insomnia; relieves menstrual cramps.	Drink 1 to 3 cups infusion daily, or take 1 to 2 droppersful tincture twice daily.	No safety concerns known	
St. John's wort *Hypericum perforatum*	Reduces skin inflammation (external use); treats mild to moderate depression and eases nerve pain (internal use).	Apply oil liberally to affected areas 1 or 2 times daily (external use); take 2 droppersful tincture twice daily (internal use); many commercial preparations available.	Do not use without the advice of an expert or experienced herbalist	
Stevia, sweet leaf *Stevia rebaudiana*	Serves as a nonnutritive sweetener; helps fight tooth decay.	Add to food and drink as desired.	Considered safe	
Thyme *Thymus vulgaris*	Acts as an antibiotic for upper respiratory tract infections and coughs (internal use); treats fungal infections (external use).	Drink 1/2 to 1 cup infusion up to 3 times daily (internal use); apply diluted oil as needed (external use).	Not recommended, especially internal use of the oil	
Turmeric *Curcuma longa*	Promotes good digestion; reduces inflammation; helps prevent diseases like cancer and heart disease when used long-term.	Drink 2 to 3 cups infusion daily, or take 1 to 2 droppersful tincture or 3 capsules or tablets, 2 or 3 times daily; use in cooking.	Considered safe	
Valerian *Valeriana officinalis*	Calms and eases anxiety and insomnia.	Take 2 to 3 droppersful of the tincture twice daily, especially before bedtime.	No safety concerns known at recommended doses; consult an experienced practitioner for higher doses	
Vitex *Vitex agnus-castus*	Eases symptoms of PMS, such as breast tenderness; balances progesterone and other sex hormones.	Take 1 to 2 droppersful tincture 1 or 2 times daily, or 1 or 2 capsules or tablets daily.	Do not use without the advice of an expert or experienced herbalist	
Wormwood *Artemisia absinthium*	Eases digestive discomfort; promotes healthy appetite; reduces nausea; treats intestinal parasites.	Drink 1/2 to 1 cup infusion before meals.	Not recommended	
Yarrow *Achillea millefolium*	Eases symptoms of colds, flu, painful digestion, PMS (especially cramping), poor fat digestion, and a feeling of fullness after meals; reduces fever and inflammation.	Drink 1 cup infusion or take 1 to 2 droppersful tincture, 2 or 3 times daily.	Not recommended	
Yerba mansa *Anemopsis californica*	Acts as an antiviral and decongestant for respiratory tract infections, colds, and flu; treats sore throats, urinary tract infections, and diarrhea.	Take 1 to 2 droppersful tincture or drink 1/2 to 1 cup decoction, 2 or 3 times daily.	Not recommended	

| | CAN BE USED IN | | | | | | | |
Infusions	Decoctions	Dried Teas	Bath Teas	Syrups	Tinctures	Oils	Compresses	Creams, Lotions, and Salves
Yes		Yes	Yes	Yes	Yes		Yes	Yes
Yes				Yes	Yes			
Yes		Yes			Yes	Yes	Yes	Yes
Yes		Yes		Yes	Yes			Yes
Yes				Yes				Yes
	Yes	Yes			Yes	Yes	Yes	Yes
Yes, 30 minutes steep time		Yes		Yes	Yes	Yes		
Yes, 30 minutes steep time		Yes			Yes			
Yes								
Yes			Yes		Yes	Yes	Yes	Yes
Yes, 30 minutes steep time		Yes		Yes	Yes	Yes	Yes	

RESOURCES

Education

Bastyr University
www.bastyr.edu

California School of Herbal Studies
www.cshs.com

East West School of Planetary Herbology
www.planetherbs.com

Foundations of Herbalism
www.foundationsofherbalism.com

North American Institute of Medical Herbalism, Inc.
www.naimh.com

Sage Mountain Retreat Center and Botanical Sanctuary
www.sagemountain.com

Tai Sophia Institute
www.tai.edu

Information

American Botanical Council
www.herbalgram.org

American Herb Association
www.ahaherb.com

American Herbal Products Association
www.ahpa.org

American Herbalists Guild
www.americanherbalist.com

Dr. Duke's Phytochemical and Ethnobotanical Database
www.ars-grin.gov/duke

Herb Growing and Marketing Network
www.herbworld.com

Herb Research Foundation
www.herbs.org

Herb Society of America
www.herbsociety.org

Local Herbs
www.localherbs.org

Plants for a Future
www.pfaf.org

United Plant Savers
www.unitedplantsavers.org

Seeds, Plants, and Garden Information and Products

Companion Plants
www.companionplants.com

Crimson Sage Medicinal Plants Nursery
www.crimson-sage.com

Gardener's Supply Company
www.gardeners.com

Goodwin Creek Gardens
www.goodwincreekgardens.com

Harmony Farm Supply and Nursery
www.harmonyfarm.com

Horizon Herbs
www.horizonherbs.com

Jean's Greens Herbal Tea Works and Herbal Essentials
www.jeansgreens.com

Nichols Garden Nursery
www.nicholsgardennursery.com

Organic Farming Research Foundation
www.ofrf.org

Peaceful Valley Farm Supply
www.groworganic.com

Plants of the Southwest
www.plantsofthesouthwest.com

Richters Herbs
www.richters.com

Products and Suppliers

Asia Natural Products, Inc.
www.drkangformulas.com

Avena Botanicals
www.avenaherbs.com

Chinese Medicinal Herb Farm
www.chinesemedicinalherbfarm.com

The Essential Oil Company
www.essentialoil.com

Frontier Natural Products Co-op
www.frontiercoop.com

Fungi Perfecti
www.fungi.com

Healing Spirits Herb Farm and Education Center
www.healingspiritsherbfarm.com

Herb Pharm
www.herb-pharm.com

Herbalist and Alchemist
www.herbalist-alchemist.com

Mayway
www.mayway.com

Mountain Rose Herbs
www.mountainroseherbs.com

Pacific Botanicals
www.pacificbotanicals.com

Rainbow Light Nutritional Systems
www.rainbowlight.com

Starwest Botanicals
www.starwest-botanicals.com

Medicine Making Supplies

AliExpress (dehydrators)
www.aliexpress.com

California Glass (bottles, jars, containers)
www.calglass.com

Harvest Essentials (dehydrators, juicers, blenders, canning supplies)
www.harvestessentials.com

Miracle Exclusives (juicers, cooking and processing tools)
www.miracleexclusives.net

INDEX

Underscored page references indicate sidebars and tables. **Boldface** references indicate photographs.

A

Acanthaceae. *See* Andrographis
Achillea millefolium. See
    Yarrow
Acidity, soil, 109–10
Acne, 185–86, 203
  herbs treating
    aloe vera, 3
    burdock, 19
    elder, 37
    honeysuckle, 47
    Oregon grape, 70, 71
    red clover, 75
    vitex, 97
Acupressure, for treating
    nausea, 199
Adaptogens
  during cancer treatment,
    59
  for treating
    diabetes, 186
    fatigue, 189
    hypertension, 194
    menopause, 196
    nervousness, 201
    premenstrual syndrome,
      202, 203
    stress, 13, 17, 77, 206
    ulcers, 207, 208
Adoxaceae. *See* Elder;
    Honeysuckle
Agastache foeniculum. See Anise
    hyssop
Agricultural fabric, 111–12
Air circulation, for drying herbs,
    132
Alcohol, for tinctures, 165–66
Alcohol use, liver health and,
    195
Alfalfa, for high cholesterol,
    183

Alkalinity, soil, 109–10
Allergies
  mucus congestion with,
    197
  sinus flushing for, 198
  skin ailments from, 203
Allium sativum. See Garlic
Aloe vera, **2**
  conditions treated by, 3
    burns, 182
    constipation, 184
    digestive problems, 188
    heartburn, 192
    high cholesterol, 183
    skin ailments, 186, 203
    ulcers, 207
    urinary tract infections,
      209
  for diabetes management,
    186
  growing, 136–37
  for liver health, 195
  profile of, 2–3, 210–11
Aloysia citriodora. See Lemon
    verbena
Aloysia triphylla. See Lemon
    verbena
Althaea officinalis. See
    Marshmallow
Amaryllidaceae. *See* Garlic
American ginseng, for stress
    reduction, 206
Andrographis, **4**
  conditions treated by, 5
    colds and flu, 184
    urinary tract infections,
      209
  growing, 136–37
  profile of, 4–5, 210–11
Andrographis paniculata. See
    Andrographis
Anemopsis californica. See Yerba
    mansa

Angelica, **6**
  conditions treated by, 7
    constipation, 184
    digestive problems, 187
    fatigue, 189
    menopause, 196
    mucus congestion, 198
    skin ailments, 204
  growing, 136–37
  profile of, 6–7, 210–11
Angelica archangelica. See
    Angelica
Anise hyssop, **8**
  conditions treated by, 9
    digestive problems,
      187
    sore throat, 205
  for gas prevention, 191
  growing, 136–37
  profile of, 8–9, 210–11
Anthemis nobilis. See
    Chamomile
Antifungal Cream, 176
Anxiety, 200–201
  herbs treating
    California poppy, 23
    gotu kola, 42, 43
    hawthorn, 45
    rhodiola, 77
    skullcap, 85
    St. John's wort, 89
    tulsi, 17
    valerian, 95
Apiaceae. *See* Angelica;
    Fennel; Gotu kola
Arctium lappa. See Burdock
Artemisia absinthium. See
    Wormwood
Arthritis, 170, 181
  herbs treating
    ashwagandha, 13
    burdock, 19
    cayenne, 27

DISCARD